Neonatal Screening for Critical Congenital Heart Defects

Neonatal Screening for Critical Congenital Heart Defects

Special Issue Editor
Andrew Ewer

MDPI • Basel • Beijing • Wuhan • Barcelona • Belgrade

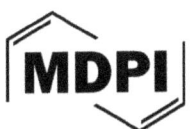

Special Issue Editor
Andrew Ewer
University of Birmingham
UK

Editorial Office
MDPI
St. Alban-Anlage 66
4052 Basel, Switzerland

This is a reprint of articles from the Special Issue published online in the open access journal *International Journal of Neonatal Screening* (ISSN 2409-515X) from 2018 to 2019 (available at: https://www.mdpi.com/journal/IJNS/special_issues/cchd)

For citation purposes, cite each article independently as indicated on the article page online and as indicated below:

LastName, A.A.; LastName, B.B.; LastName, C.C. Article Title. *Journal Name* **Year**, *Article Number*, Page Range.

ISBN 978-3-03921-048-0 (Pbk)
ISBN 978-3-03921-049-7 (PDF)

© 2019 by the authors. Articles in this book are Open Access and distributed under the Creative Commons Attribution (CC BY) license, which allows users to download, copy and build upon published articles, as long as the author and publisher are properly credited, which ensures maximum dissemination and a wider impact of our publications.

The book as a whole is distributed by MDPI under the terms and conditions of the Creative Commons license CC BY-NC-ND.

Contents

About the Special Issue Editor vii

Andrew K. Ewer
Pulse Oximetry Screening for Critical Congenital Heart Defects: A Life-Saving Test for All Newborn Babies
Reprinted from: *Int. J. Neonatal Screen.* **2019**, *5*, 14, doi:10.3390/ijns5010014 1

Scott D. Grosse, Cora Peterson, Rahi Abouk, Jill Glidewell and Matthew E. Oster
Cost and Cost-Effectiveness Assessments of Newborn Screening for Critical Congenital Heart Disease Using Pulse Oximetry: A Review
Reprinted from: *Int. J. Neonatal Screen.* **2017**, *3*, 34, doi:10.3390/ijns3040034 7

Martin Kluckow
Barriers to the Implementation of Newborn Pulse Oximetry Screening: A Different Perspective
Reprinted from: *Int. J. Neonatal Screen.* **2018**, *4*, 4, doi:10.3390/ijns4010004 22

Thomas L. Gentles, Elza Cloete and Mats Mellander
Comment on Kluckow M. Barriers to the Implementation of Newborn Pulse Oximetry Screening: A Different Perspective. *Int. J. Neonatal Screen.* 2018, 4(1), 4
Reprinted from: *Int. J. Neonatal Screen.* **2018**, *4*, 13, doi:10.3390/ijns4020013 29

Martin Kluckow
A Reply to Comment on Kluckow M. Barriers to the Implementation of Newborn Pulse Oximetry Screening: A Different Perspective. *Int. J. Neonatal Screen.* 2018, 4(1), 4
Reprinted from: *Int. J. Neonatal Screen.* **2018**, *4*, 14, doi:10.3390/ijns4020014 31

Ilona C. Narayen, Nico A. Blom and Arjan B. te Pas
Pulse Oximetry Screening Adapted to a System with Home Births: The Dutch Experience
Reprinted from: *Int. J. Neonatal Screen.* **2018**, *4*, 11, doi:10.3390/ijns4020011 32

Frank-Thomas Riede, Christian Paech and Thorsten Orlikowsky
Pulse Oximetry Screening in Germany—Historical Aspects and Future Perspectives
Reprinted from: *Int. J. Neonatal Screen.* **2018**, *4*, 15, doi:10.3390/ijns4020015 38

Lisa A. Wandler and Gerard R. Martin
Critical Congenital Heart Disease Screening Using Pulse Oximetry: Achieving a National Approach to Screening, Education and Implementation in the United States
Reprinted from: *Int. J. Neonatal Screen.* **2017**, *3*, 28, doi:10.3390/ijns3040028 47

William Walsh and Jean A. Ballweg
A Single-Extremity Staged Approach for Critical Congenital Heart Disease Screening: Results from Tennessee
Reprinted from: *Int. J. Neonatal Screen.* **2017**, *3*, 31, doi:10.3390/ijns3040031 58

Elena Cubells, Begoña Torres, Antonio Nuñez-Ramiro, Manuel Sánchez-Luna, Isabel Izquierdo and Máximo Vento
Congenital Critical Heart Defect Screening in a Health Area of the Community of Valencia (Spain): A Prospective Observational Study
Reprinted from: *Int. J. Neonatal Screen.* **2018**, *4*, 3, doi:10.3390/ijns4010003 63

Augusto Sola and Sergio G. Golombek
Early Detection with Pulse Oximetry of Hypoxemic Neonatal Conditions. Development of the IX Clinical Consensus Statement of the Ibero-American Society of Neonatology (SIBEN)
Reprinted from: *Int. J. Neonatal Screen.* **2018**, *4*, 10, doi:10.3390/ijns4010010 . . . . **69**

John S. Kim, Merlin W. Ariefdjohan, Marci K. Sontag and Christopher M. Rausch
Pulse Oximetry Values in Newborns with Critical Congenital Heart Disease upon ICU Admission at Altitude
Reprinted from: *Int. J. Neonatal Screen.* **2018**, *4*, 30, doi:10.3390/ijns4040030 . . . . **79**

About the Special Issue Editor

Andrew Ewer is Professor of Neonatal Medicine at the University of Birmingham and Honorary Consultant Neonatologist at Birmingham Women's Hospital. He qualified from Birmingham (UK) and trained in Paediatrics and Neonatology in Birmingham (UK), Sheffield (UK) and Melbourne (Australia). He was awarded MD in 1998. He led the HTA-funded PulseOx study between 2007 and 2011, which investigated test accuracy, health economics and the acceptability of pulse oximetry screening. He has published widely on pulse oximetry screening, including 3 systematic reviews (2007 [ADCFN] 2012 [Lancet] and 2018 [Cochrane library]). He advised the USA SACHDNC (the Secretary's Advisory Committee on Heritable Disorders in Newborns and Children) committee prior to the introduction of screening for critical congenital heart defects in January 2011. He has worked with NIPE/NSC (the NHS newborn and infant physical examination/ National Screening Committee) UK since 2011 and was clinical lead for the UK pulse oximetry screening pilot study in 2015. He is a senior member of the European Workgroup on pulse oximetry screening, and published a European consensus statement in 2017. In the last five years, he has given over 30 overseas lectures across five continents and advised numerous organizations and countries regarding the introduction of screening.

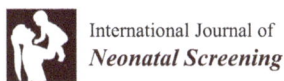 International Journal of
Neonatal Screening

Editorial

Pulse Oximetry Screening for Critical Congenital Heart Defects: A Life-Saving Test for All Newborn Babies

Andrew K. Ewer [1,2]

1. Institute of Metabolism and Systems Research, University of Birmingham, Birmingham B15 2TT, UK; a.k.ewer@bham.ac.uk
2. Neonatal Unit, Birmingham Women's and Children's Hospital NHS Foundation Trust, Birmingham B15 2TG, UK

Received: 31 January 2019; Accepted: 11 February 2019; Published: 12 February 2019

Congenital heart defects (CHD) are the commonest congenital malformations and remain a major cause of neonatal mortality and morbidity in the developed world [1,2]. Critical congenital heart defects (CCHD) are the most serious form of CHD, with an incidence of between two and three per 1000 live births [3]. Babies with CCHD are at risk of cardiovascular collapse, acidosis, and death in the first few days of life, usually following closure of the ductus arteriosus; therefore, early diagnosis is essential to reduce the possibility of these complications and also to improve outcomes following cardiac surgery [1,2].

In high-income countries, most babies are routinely screened for CCHD using antenatal ultrasound scanning and postnatal physical examination. However, both of these procedures have a relatively low detection rate, and up to a third of babies with CCHD may be discharged from hospital before a diagnosis is made [4,5].

Pulse oximetry (PO) measures blood oxygen saturations and is a well-established, accurate, non-invasive method of detecting low oxygen levels (hypoxaemia) [1,2]. The rationale for using PO to screen for CCHD is that hypoxaemia is present in the majority of cases of CCHD, but the degree of desaturation is often comparatively mild and may be clinically undetectable, even by experienced clinicians [6]. Therefore, the addition of PO screening (POS) following delivery will detect those babies with hypoxaemia, who can then be assessed and the presence of a CCHD established before the babies develop acute collapse [1].

Proof of concept and feasibility of POS was first established by a number of small single centre studies in the early 2000s, but the low prevalence of CCHD in these studies meant that there was insufficient evidence to precisely define the test accuracy, and firm recommendations for routine screening could not be made [2,7]. Between 2008 and 2012, several large European studies provided sufficient, robust evidence of test accuracy which could reliably inform the possible introduction of routine POS [8–12].

In 2012, a systematic review and meta-analysis of all available evidence (including nearly 230,000 screened babies) concluded that pulse oximetry screening was a moderately sensitive, highly specific test for detection of CCHD, which met the criteria for universal screening [13]. In 2014, the world's largest POS study involving over 120,000 babies from China [14] demonstrated similar findings which essentially removed any remaining uncertainties about the performance of PO screening [15].

The addition of POS reduces the 'diagnostic gap' for CCHD [10] (i.e. those babies who are not detected by existing screening methods), and when POS is combined with antenatal ultrasound scanning and the newborn physical examination, between 92% and 96% of babies with CCHD are identified in a timely manner [16].

Attitudes towards POS are changing, and acceptance of the potential benefits is becoming more widespread. In 2012, a Lancet editorial commented '... surely, the question now is not "why should pulse oximetry screening be introduced?" but "why should such screening not be introduced more widely?"' [17]. The papers within this special edition book for the *International Journal of Neonatal Screening* address many of the broader aspects of POS beyond the basic test accuracy; topics include acceptability, cost-effectiveness, screening in different settings—such as outside the newborn nursery environment and at altitude—and, importantly, implementation of POS in different countries and clinical settings and establishing a screening system which suits the local population.

Giving appropriate information and assessing the acceptability of any screening test—both to the patients involved and to the clinical staff who administer it—is vital if it is to be successful. Previous studies have shown that POS is acceptable to parents and clinical staff [12,18,19] and also that it does not appear to create additional anxiety in the mothers (including those who have a false positive result) [18]. In this special edition, Cloete et al. report feedback from parents on both the information they received prior to testing and their overall satisfaction of POS during a pilot screening study in New Zealand [20]. The cultural diversity and the mainly midwifery-led maternity system in this country make the positive responses received particularly pertinent. As part of their extensive overview of the implementation process of POS in the USA—the first country to legislate for mandatory POS of all newborns—Wandler and Martin also report on their systematic and highly effective approach to addressing the issues raised by such a huge undertaking [21].

As well as being acceptable, a new screening test must also be shown to be cost-effective. A number of previous studies in different countries have tried to address this issue [9,22–24].

In their review of this work in this special edition, Scott Grosse and colleagues provide a comprehensive analysis of the available evidence, including a revised estimate of cost (based on recent improved survival figures from the US following the introduction of POS), estimating that the cost could be as low as USD 12,000 per life-year gained [25].

Switzerland, Ireland, and Poland were the first countries to recommend routine POS [16,26], and in 2011, as described above, the USA was the first country to mandate this test [27,28].

Over the past five years, an increasing number of countries, including Canada [29], the Nordic countries [30], Saudi Arabia, Abu Dhabi, and Sri Lanka [26], have recommended routine screening. In Europe, significant progress has been made by a multinational group of clinicians working towards a Europe-wide implementation of PO screening [31] and recently publishing a European consensus statement, endorsed by leading figures from European Paediatric and Neonatal Societies [32]. In this special edition, further national recommendations are published from Germany [33] and South and Central America [34], in addition to a local study from Valencia, Spain [35], which was one of the precursors to the recent Spanish recommendation [36]. In the UK, almost half of all maternity units are screening [37] but there is no national recommendation as yet. In Australia, a different approach has been taken; in this special edition, Martin Kluckow suggests that pulse oximetry should be considered a 'routine vital sign' of general neonatal wellbeing rather than a test for a specific target such as CCHD [38]. This allows individual hospitals to screen in a manner which suits them and might make the process simpler and potentially more acceptable; this is an approach which seems to have worked in Australia, but in response, Gentles et al. argue that a structured national recommendation would ensure a more equitable service to the whole population [39]. Kluckow's reply highlights the fact that national recommendations are often rather slow and cumbersome and that babies may miss out on screening until the recommendation is sanctioned [40].

Screening pathways (or algorithms) for POS within the published studies are variable [7,13,41,42]. The main differences are i) site of saturation measurement (the use of a single [post-ductal] saturation measurement or measuring both pre- and post-ductal saturations) and ii) the timing of screening (before or after 24 h of age).

Screening algorithms which use only a single post-ductal measurement are potentially quicker and easier, but investigation of the data from these studies and those using both pre- and post-ductal saturations show that a small number of babies with CCHD may be missed by using only a single post-ductal measurement [16,41,42]. With large populations, this number may become significant, and the benefits of using two measurements may outweigh the potential minor disadvantages [16,40,42]. Most of the recent recommendations advocate dual site measurements, but Riede and colleagues recommend post-ductal saturation measurement only [33]. An interesting alternative strategy is proposed by Walsh and Ballweg from Tennessee USA, who advocate post-ductal saturations with a higher threshold (97%) for the initial screen and then pre- and post-ductal saturations for those who require a repeat [43].

As with any screening test, it is important to consider the number of false positives (those babies who have a positive test but do not have CCHD), and the timing of the PO screen affects the number of false positive screens [13,41]. Later screening (>24 hours) has a lower rate of false positive tests [13,41]; however, between 30% and 80% of false positive babies have a significant respiratory or infective condition or non-critical CHD [16,25,42,44]. Earlier screening is mandatory in countries (such as the UK where the majority of babies are discharged within 24 h after birth or in the Netherlands where many babies are born outside of the hospital environment). In addition, screening after 24 h of age may result in up to half of babies with CCHD presenting before POS occurs, sometimes with an acute deterioration [16,42]. These factors must be considered carefully; although a lower number of false positives is advantageous in a screening test, if the majority of false positives have a serious non-cardiac condition which requires urgent treatment, this is clearly a significant additional benefit [19]. In addition, later screening—after 24 hours—may lead to more babies with CCHD becoming seriously unwell before testing takes place, which defeats the purpose of screening [16,42]. As more countries engage with POS and high-quality outcome data are collected, the nuances of modifying and refining the screening algorithms can be modelled with greater precision [42].

Screening babies born outside of the nursery e.g., at home, in a midwifery-led birthing centre, or on the neonatal intensive care unit (NICU), present particular challenges; with homebirth midwifery staff often leave the mother and baby shortly after birth, which means that POS must take place within a couple of hours. However, screening babies in this situation has been shown to be both feasible and acceptable in a small UK study [45] and a much larger Dutch study [46,47]. In this special edition, Narayen and colleagues present their experience screening such babies in the Netherlands [48] and Kim et al. report their findings of screening newborns on the NICU at moderate altitude (1700m) [49].

In summary, PO screening is feasible, cost-effective, and acceptable, and it also reduces the diagnostic gap for CCHD. This special edition of the *International Journal of Neonatal Screening* focuses on a number of issues which are entirely relevant to those who might be considering introducing such screening.

A universal programme of PO screening in newborns will increase the detection of CCHD, and importantly, it has also been shown to be useful in identifying other potentially life-threatening clinical conditions (such as respiratory problems and sepsis), which is an important additional advantage. In a very important report from the USA, Abouk et al. report a 33% reduction in mortality from CCHD in US states that had introduced POS compared with those where introduction had not yet occurred [50].

When defining the most appropriate screening algorithm, a balance must be struck between detection of a serious illness and limiting false positive results, and local circumstances may play a role in this respect. More data from larger populations may help to refine further the screening algorithm. Finally, it is also important to remember that PO screening is not a perfect test, and babies with CCHD may still be missed [15,16]. Therefore, PO screening should be used as an addition to existing screening methods, and health care workers and parents need to be aware of the limitations of the test.

Conflicts of Interest: The authors declare no conflict of interest.

References

1. Ewer, A.K.; Furmston, A.T.; Middleton, L.J. Pulse oximetry as a screening test for congenital heart defects in newborn infants: A test accuracy study with evaluation of acceptability and cost-effectiveness. *Health Technol. Assess.* **2012**, *16*, 1–184. [CrossRef] [PubMed]

2. Mahle, W.T.; Newburger, J.W.; Matherne, G.P.; Smith, F.C.; Hoke, T.R.; Koppel, R. Role of pulse oximetry in examining newborns for congenital heart disease: A scientific statement from the AHA and AAP. *Pediatrics* **2009**, *124*, 823–836. [CrossRef] [PubMed]
3. Hoffman, J.I.E.; Kaplan, S. The incidence of congenital heart disease. *J. Am. Coll. Cardiol.* **2002**, *39*, 1890–1900. [CrossRef]
4. Wren, C.; Reinhardt, Z.; Khawaja, K. Twenty-year trends in diagnosis of life-threatening neonatal cardiovascular malformations. *Arch. Dis. Child. Fetal Neonatal. Ed.* **2008**, *93*, F33–F35. [CrossRef] [PubMed]
5. Acharya, G.; Sitras, V.; Maltau, J.M.; Dahl, L.B.; Kaaresen, P.I.; Hanssen, T.A. Major congenital heart disease in Northern Norway: Shortcomings of pre- and postnatal diagnosis. *Acta Obstet. Gynecol. Scand.* **2004**, *83*, 1124–1129. [CrossRef] [PubMed]
6. O'Donnell, C.P.F.; Kamlin, C.O.F.; Davis, P.G.; Carlin, J.B.; Morley, C.J. Clinical assessment of infant colour at delivery. *Arch. Dis. Child. Fetal Neonatal. Ed.* **2007**, *92*, F465–F467. [CrossRef] [PubMed]
7. Thangaratinam, S.; Daniels, J.; Ewer, A.K.; Zamora, J.; Khan, K.S. The accuracy of pulse oximetry in screening for congenital heart disease in asymptomatic newborns: A systematic review. *Arch. Dis. Child. Fetal Neonatal. Ed.* **2007**, *92*, F176–F180. [CrossRef] [PubMed]
8. Meberg, A.; Brugmann-Pieper, S.; Eskedal, L.; Fagerli, I.; Farstad, T. First day of life pulse oximetry screening to detect congenital heart defects. *J. Pediatr.* **2008**, *152*, 761–765. [CrossRef] [PubMed]
9. De-Wahl Granelli, A.; Wennergren, M.; Sandberg, K. Impact of pulse oximetry screening on the detection of duct dependent congenital heart disease: A Swedish prospective screening study in 39,821 newborns. *BMJ* **2009**, *338*, a3037. [CrossRef] [PubMed]
10. Riede, F.T.; Worner, C.; Dahnert, I. Effectiveness of neonatal pulse oximetry screening for detection of critical congenital heart disease in daily clinical routine: Results from a prospective multicenter study. *Eur J. Pediatr.* **2010**, *169*, 975–981. [CrossRef] [PubMed]
11. Ewer, A.K.; Middleton, L.J.; Furmston, A.T.; Bhoyar, A.; Daniels, J.P.; Thangaratinam, S.; Deeks, J.J.; Khan, K.S. Pulse oximetry as a screening test for congenital heart defects in newborn infants (PulseOx): A test accuracy study. *Lancet* **2011**, *378*, 785–794. [CrossRef]
12. Turska Kmieć, A.; Borszewska Kornacka, M.K.; Błaż, W. Early screening for critical congenital heart defects in asymptomatic newborns in Mazovia province: Experience of the POLKARD pulse oximetry programme 2006–2008 in Poland. *Kardiol. Polska* **2012**, *70*, 370–376.
13. Thangaratinam, S.; Daniels J Ewer, A.K.; Zamora, J.; Khan, K.S. Pulse oximetry screening for critical congenital heart defects in asymptomatic newborn babies: A systematic review and meta-analysis. *Lancet* **2012**, *379*, 2459–2464. [CrossRef]
14. Zhao, Q.; Ma, X.; Ge, X. Using Pulse Oximetry Combined with Clinical Evaluation to Screen Congenital Heart Disease in Early Neonatal Stage: A Chinese prospective screening study in 122,738 newborns. *Lancet* **2014**, *384*, 747–754. [CrossRef]
15. Ewer, A.K. Pulse oximetry screening: Do we have enough evidence now? *Lancet* **2014**, *384*, 725–726. [CrossRef]
16. Ewer, A.K. Review of pulse oximetry screening for critical congenital heart defects. *Curr. Opin. Cardiol.* **2013**, *28*, 92–96. [CrossRef] [PubMed]
17. The Lancet. A new milestone in the history of congenital heart disease. *Lancet* **2012**, *379*, 2401. [CrossRef]
18. Powell, R.; Pattison, H.M.; Bhoyar, A. Pulse oximetry as a screening test for congenital heart defects in newborn infants: An evaluation of acceptability to mothers. *Arch. Dis. Child. Fetal Neonatal. Ed.* **2013**, *98*, F59–F63. [CrossRef] [PubMed]
19. Narayen, I.C.; Kaptein, A.A.; Hogewoning, J.A.; Blom, N.A.; te Pas, A.B. Maternal acceptability of pulse oximetry screening at home after home birth or very early discharge. *Eur. J. Pediatr.* **2017**, *176*, 669–672. [CrossRef] [PubMed]
20. Cloete, E.; Gentles, T.L.; Lutter, R.A.; Richards, K.; Ward, K.; Bloomfield, F.H. Consumer satisfaction with newborn pulse oximetry screening in a midwifery-led maternity setting. *Int. J. Neonatal Screen.* **2018**, *4*, 38. [CrossRef]
21. Wandler, L.A.; Martin, G.R. Critical congenital heart disease screening using pulse Oximetry: Achieving a national approach to screening, education and implementation in the United States. *Int. J. Neonatal Screen.* **2017**, *3*, 28. [CrossRef]

22. Roberts, T.E.; Barton, P.; Auguste, P. Pulse oximetry as a screening test for congenital heart disease in newborn infants: A cost effectiveness analysis. *Arch. Dis. Child.* **2012**, *97*, 221–226. [CrossRef] [PubMed]
23. Peterson, C.; Grosse, S.D.; Oster, M.E.; Olney, R.S.; Cassell, C.H. Cost-effectiveness of routine screening for Critical Congenital Heart Disease in US newborns. *Pediatrics* **2013**, *132*, e595. [CrossRef] [PubMed]
24. Kochilas, L.K.; Lohr, J.L.; Bruhn, E.; Borman-Shoap, E. Implementation of critical congenital heart disease screening in Minnesota. *Pediatrics* **2013**, *132*, e587–e594. [CrossRef] [PubMed]
25. Grosse, S.D.; Peterson, C.; Abouk, R.; Glidewell, J.; Oster, M.E. Cost and Cost-Effectiveness Assessments of Newborn Screening for Critical Congenital Heart Disease Using Pulse Oximetry: A Review. *Int. J. Neonatal Screen.* **2017**, *3*, 34. [CrossRef] [PubMed]
26. Narayen, I.C.; Blom, N.A.; Ewer, A.K.; Vento, M.; Manzoni, P.; te Pas, A.B. Aspects of pulse oximetry screening for critical congenital heart defects: When, how and why. *Arch. Dis. Child. Fetal Neonatal. Ed.* **2015**. [CrossRef] [PubMed]
27. Kemper, A.R.; Mahle, W.T.; Martin, G.R.; Cooley, W.C.; Kumar, P.; Morrow, W.R. Strategies for implementing screening for critical congenital heart disease. *Pediatrics* **2011**, *128*, e1259–e1267. [CrossRef] [PubMed]
28. Mahle, W.T.; Martin, G.R.; Beekman, R.H. Endorsement of Health and Human Services recommendation for pulse oximetry screening for critical congenital heart disease. *Pediatrics.* **2012**, *129*, 190–192. [PubMed]
29. Wong, K.K.; Fournier, A.; Fruitman, D.S.; Graves, L. Canadian Cardiovascular Society/Canadian Pediatric Cardiology Association Position Statement on Pulse Oximetry Screening in Newborns to Enhance Detection of Critical Congenital Heart Disease. *Can. J. Cardiol.* **2017**, *33*, 199–208. [CrossRef] [PubMed]
30. De-Wahl Granelli, A.; Meberg, A.; Ojala, T.; Steensberg, J.; Oskarsson, G.; Mellander, M. Nordic pulse oximetry screening–implementation status and proposal for uniform guidelines. *Acta Paediatr.* **2014**, *103*, 1136–1142. [CrossRef] [PubMed]
31. Ewer, A.K.; Granelli, A.; Manzoni, P.; Sánchez Luna, M.; Martin, G.R. Pulse Oximetry screening for critical congenital heart defects. *Lancet* **2013**, *382*, 856–857. [CrossRef]
32. Manzoni, P.; Martin, G.R.; Sanchez Luna, M.; Mestrovic, J.; Simeoni, U.; Zimmermann, L.J.I. Pulse oximetry screening for critical congenital heart defects: A European consensus statement. *Lancet Child Adolesc. Health* **2017**, *1*, 88–90. [CrossRef]
33. Riede, F.-T.; Paech, C.; Orlikowsky, T. Pulse Oximetry Screening in Germany—Historical Aspects and Future Perspectives. *Int. J. Neonatal Screen.* **2018**, *4*, 15. [CrossRef]
34. Sola, A.; Golombek, S.G. Early Detection with Pulse Oximetry of Hypoxemic Neonatal Conditions. Development of the IX Clinical Consensus Statement of the Ibero-American Society of Neonatology (SIBEN). *Int. J. Neonatal Screen.* **2018**, *4*, 10. [CrossRef]
35. Cubells, E.; Torres, B.; Nuñez-Ramiro, A.; Sánchez-Luna, M.; Izquierdo I Vento, M. Congenital critical heart defect screening in a health area of the community of Valencia (Spain): A prospective observational study. *Int. J. Neonatal Screen.* **2018**, *4*, 3. [CrossRef]
36. Sánchez Luna, M.; Pérez Muñuzuri, A.; López, E.S.; Castellanos, J.L. Pulse oximetry screening of critical congenital heart defects in the neonatal period. The Spanish National Neonatal Society recommendation. *An. Pediatr.* **2018**, *88*, e1–e112. [CrossRef]
37. Mikrou, P.; Singh, A.; Ewer, A.K. Pulse oximetry screening for critical congenital heart defects: A repeat UK national survey. *Arch. Dis. Child. Fetal Neonatal Ed.* **2017**. [CrossRef] [PubMed]
38. Kluckow, M. Barriers to the implementation of newborn pulse oximetry screening: A different perspective. *Int. J. Neonatal Screen.* **2018**, *4*, 4. [CrossRef]
39. Gentles, T.L.; Cloete, E.; Mellander, M. Comment on Kluckow M. Barriers to the Implementation of Newborn Pulse Oximetry Screening: A Different Perspective. *Int. J. Neonatal Screen.* **2018**, *4*, 13. [CrossRef]
40. Kluckow, M. A Reply to Comment on Kluckow M. Barriers to the implementation of newborn pulse oximetry screening: A different perspective. *Int. J. Neonatal Screen.* **2018**, *4*, 13. [CrossRef]
41. Plana, M.N.; Zamora, J.; Suresh, G.; Fernandez-Pineda, L.; Thangaratinam, S.; Ewer, A.K. Pulse oximetry screening for critical congenital heart defects. *Cochrane Database Syst. Rev.* **2018**. [CrossRef] [PubMed]
42. Ewer, A.K.; Martin, G.R. Newborn pulse oximetry screening: Which algorithm is best? *Pediatrics* **2016**, *138*, e20161206. [CrossRef] [PubMed]
43. Walsh, W.; Ballweg, J.A. A single-extremity staged approach for critical congenital heart disease screening: Results from Tennessee. *Int. J. Neonatal Screen.* **2017**, *3*, 31. [CrossRef]

44. Singh, A.S.; Rasiah, S.V.; Ewer, A.K. The impact of routine pre-discharge pulse oximetry screening in a regional neonatal unit. *Arch. Dis. Child. Fetal Neonatal. Ed.* **2014**, *99*, F297–F302. [CrossRef] [PubMed]
45. Cawsey, M.J.; Noble, S.; Cross-Sudworth, F.; Ewer, A.K. Feasibility of pulse oximetry screening for critical congenital heart defects in homebirths. *Arch. Dis. Child. Fetal Neonatal. Ed.* **2016**. [CrossRef] [PubMed]
46. Narayen, I.C.; Blom, N.A.; Verhart, M.S. Adapted protocol for pulse oximetry screening for congenital heart defects in a country with homebirths. *Eur J. Pediatr.* **2015**, *174*, 129–132. [CrossRef] [PubMed]
47. Narayen, I.C.; Blom, N.A.; Geloven, N.; Blankman, E.I.M. Accuracy of Pulse Oximetry Screening for Critical Congenital Heart Defects after Home Birth and Early Postnatal Discharge. *J. Pediatr.* **2018**, *197*, 29–35. [CrossRef] [PubMed]
48. Narayen, I.; Blom, N.A.; te Pas, A.B. Pulse Oximetry Screening Adapted to a System with Home Births: The Dutch Experience. *Int. J. Neonatal Screen.* **2018**, *4*, 11. [CrossRef]
49. Kim, J.S.; Ariefdjohan, M.W.; Sontag MK Rausch, C.M. Pulse oximetry values in newborns with critical congenital heart disease upon ICU admission at altitude. *Int. J. Neonatal Screen.* **2018**, *4*, 30. [CrossRef]
50. Abouk, R.; Grosse, S.D.; Ailes, E.C.; Oster, M.E. Association of US state implementation of newborn screening policies for critical congenital heart disease with early infant cardiac deaths. *JAMA* **2017**, *318*, 2111–2118. [CrossRef] [PubMed]

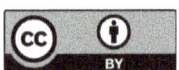

© 2019 by the author. Licensee MDPI, Basel, Switzerland. This article is an open access article distributed under the terms and conditions of the Creative Commons Attribution (CC BY) license (http://creativecommons.org/licenses/by/4.0/).

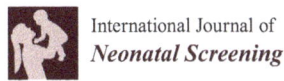

Review

Cost and Cost-Effectiveness Assessments of Newborn Screening for Critical Congenital Heart Disease Using Pulse Oximetry: A Review

Scott D. Grosse [1,*], Cora Peterson [2], Rahi Abouk [3], Jill Glidewell [1] and Matthew E. Oster [1,4]

1. Centers for Disease Control and Prevention, National Center on Birth Defects and Developmental Disabilities, 4770 Buford Highway NE, Mail Stop E-87, Atlanta, GA 30341, USA; MGlidewell@cdc.gov (J.G.); OsterM@kidsheart.com (M.E.O.)
2. Centers for Disease Control and Prevention, National Center for Injury Prevention and Control, Atlanta, GA 30341, USA; CPeterson2@cdc.gov
3. Cotsakos College of Business, William Paterson University, Wayne, NJ 07470, USA; AboukR@wpunj.edu
4. Children's Healthcare of Atlanta, Emory University School of Medicine, Atlanta, GA 30341, USA
* Correspondence: sgrosse@cdc.gov; Tel.: +1-404-498-3074

Received: 1 November 2017; Accepted: 12 December 2017; Published: 14 December 2017

Abstract: Screening newborns for critical congenital heart disease (CCHD) using pulse oximetry is recommended to allow for the prompt diagnosis and prevention of life-threatening crises. The present review summarizes and critiques six previously published estimates of the costs or cost-effectiveness of CCHD screening from the United Kingdom, United States, and China. Several elements that affect CCHD screening costs were assessed in varying numbers of studies, including screening staff time, instrumentation, and consumables, as well as costs of diagnosis and treatment. A previous US study that used conservative assumptions suggested that CCHD screening is likely to be considered cost-effective from the healthcare sector perspective. Newly available estimates of avoided infant CCHD deaths in several US states that implemented mandatory CCHD screening policies during 2011–2013 suggest a substantially larger reduction in deaths than was projected in the previous US cost-effectiveness analysis. Taking into account these new estimates, we estimate that cost per life-year gained could be as low as USD 12,000. However, that estimate does not take into account future costs of health care and education for surviving children with CCHD nor the costs incurred by health departments to support and monitor CCHD screening policies and programs.

Keywords: neonatal screening; critical congenital heart disease; economic evaluation; cost-effectiveness; health policy

---

1. Introduction

Newborn screening (NBS) can save both lives and healthcare costs, although testing for any given condition may accomplish only one or the other [1]. However, the up-front costs and logistical challenges of instituting screening of all or almost all newborn infants, few of whom will be found to be affected, can deter policy makers from instituting new screening programs or adding conditions to an existing program. The economic balance between the costs and benefits of screening has long been recognized as a desirable attribute of population screening programs [2]. Although some jurisdictions require a prospective economic assessment to inform decisions on the expansion of NBS [3], screening policy decisions have often not required a demonstration of cost-effectiveness in practice [4,5].

Although most NBS is done through centralized laboratory analyses of dried bloodspot specimens collected from newborns, point-of-care NBS for certain conditions is typically performed before discharge from the birthing facility [6]. In particular, screening for various types of critical congenital heart disease (CCHD) (Table 1) can be done using pulse oximetry, a simple, non-invasive test for hypoxemia in which sensors measure blood oxygen saturation through light passing through the skin [7]. Neonatal hypoxemia can have either cardiac or non-cardiac causes. When the US Department of Health and Human Services added CCHD to its Recommended Uniform Screening Panel in 2011, it requested the Centers for Disease Control and Prevention (CDC) to conduct a cost-effectiveness analysis (CEA) of newborn screening for CCHD [8,9]. That information was intended to inform policy decisions by state governments. In 2013, CDC researchers (Peterson et al.) published the first full CEA of CCHD screening in the US setting [10]. Although previous studies had estimated the cost of screening and the cost per case of CCHD detected [11–17], "Calculating the cost to detect a case tells one nothing about the value of detecting and treating the disease in question and, hence, is not informative of the balance of costs and outcomes" [18]. A full CEA includes estimates of the numbers of deaths averted and avoided healthcare costs associated with prompt diagnosis. Peterson et al. reported a point estimate of roughly USD 40,000 in net cost per life-year saved, a figure consistent with commonly used cost-effectiveness thresholds [19]. More recently, a CEA assessed the potential cost-effectiveness of CCHD screening in different localities in China, reporting that screening could be cost-effective in some settings [20].

Table 1. Types of Critical Congenital Heart Disease and Associated International Classification of Disease, 10th Version (ICD-10) Diagnosis Codes.

CCHD Types	ICD-10 Codes
Aortic interruption or atresia or hypoplasia	Q25.4, Q25.2
Coarctation or hypoplasia of the aortic arch	Q25.1
D-transposition of the great arteries	Q20.3
Double-outlet right ventricle	Q20.1
Ebstein anomaly	Q22.5
Hypoplastic left heart syndrome	Q23.4
Pulmonary atresia	Q22.0
Single ventricle	Q20.4
Teratology of Fallot	Q21.3
Total anomalous pulmonary venous connection	Q26.2
Tricuspid stenosis and atresia	Q22.4
Truncus arteriosus	Q20.0

The present review summarizes and critiques previously published estimates of the costs or cost-effectiveness of CCHD screening—two UK studies in four publications [12–14,17], three US studies in four publications [10,21–23], and one study from China [20]. Updated estimates of costs, outcomes, and summary measures of the economic value of CCHD screening in the United States are also presented. The new estimates address future disease-related treatment costs, shortened life expectancy among CCHD survivors, and a higher estimated number of avoided infant deaths due to screening.

2. Review of Previous Estimates

CEA studies of screening programs or policies require as inputs, estimates of the costs of screening, diagnosis, and intervention, numbers of cases detected in a timely manner as a result of screening, differences in health outcomes with and without screening (i.e., effectiveness), and differences in healthcare and other costs for affected individuals between scenarios with and without screening [18,24]. Each of those parameters is context-specific; therefore, it is difficult to use a given study to generalize as to whether screening may be cost-effective in different contexts. For example, a given screening test may have very different costs and outcomes in different settings depending on the characteristics of the population and how screening is implemented in that setting. In addition, the assessment of cost-effectiveness depends on how much decision makers are willing to pay for an intervention or program in relation to the expected health gains. This means that different stakeholders and jurisdictions that consider the same evidence on costs and outcomes may reach different conclusions about economic value. Therefore, instead of asking whether screening is cost-effective, it may be more constructive to ask when and by whom screening might be considered cost-effective [24,25].

The analytic perspective of an economic evaluation must be specified. From the societal or healthcare sector perspectives, cost refers to the opportunity cost of resources used up in providing a service rather than the direct financial outlay or expenditure of money. Many CEAs of clinical interventions take the healthcare sector (or system) perspective, in which only formal healthcare sector costs are considered [26,27]. A societal perspective analysis should also include informal healthcare costs, such as the time and expenses incurred by patients and families, non-health sector costs such as educational expenditures, and productivity losses resulting from death or premature mortality [28]. Spillover effects of illness or disability on the health of family members and on the time use and economic productivity of family caregivers are also germane for societal-perspective cost-effectiveness analyses [29]. The societal perspective is particularly appropriate for the analysis of public health policies and programs, and such analyses should include the costs of public health activities in support of clinical interventions.

2.1. Cost of Critical Congenital Heart Disease (CCHD) Screening and Follow-Up

The one element common to all previous economic evaluations of CCHD screening is inclusion of the directly estimated cost of screening, which is readily measurable for CCHD screening. Most studies employed a micro-costing approach with separate estimates for staff time, instrumentation, and consumables (Table 2). An exception is a cost-effectiveness study from China that did not report detailed screening costs [20]. The micro-costing estimates from other studies are summarized below separately for labor (Section 2.1.1) and instruments and consumables (Section 2.1.2). In addition to the direct costs of pulse oximetry screening, the incremental cost of CCHD screening includes the costs incurred by the healthcare system for the follow-up and management of patients who screen positive. That includes clinical examinations and diagnostic tests attributable to screening. It also includes the differences in treatment costs that result from early diagnosis. Estimates for those cost components are summarized in Sections 2.1.3 and 2.1.4.

Table 2. Summary of data assumptions of micro-costing studies of critical congenital heart disease screening.

Study	Country and Jurisdiction	Screening Time (Minutes)	Screening Staff Type and Labor Cost per Infant	Type of Probes, and Equipment/Supply Cost per Infant	Total Screening Cost per Infant
Knowles et al. [13,14]	United Kingdom	2.0	Senior house officer £1.54 $2.20 (USD)	Reusable £1.28 $1.83 (USD)	£2.82 (2000–2001 prices) $4.03 (USD)
Roberts et al. [12]	United Kingdom	6.9	Midwives Not reported	Reusable Not reported	£6.24 (2009 prices) $8.80 (USD)
Peterson et al. [21]	United States New Jersey	9.1	Registered nurses $7.36	Mixed types $6.83	$14.19 (2011 prices)
Kochilas et al. [22]	United States Minnesota	5.5	Nursing staff $3.32	Reusable $1.82	$5.10 (2012 prices)
Reeder er al. [23]	United States Utah (two hospitals)	8.4	Medical assistants and nurses $2.60	Disposable $21.92	$24.52 (2014 prices)
		9.8	Nursing assistants $2.35	Reusable $0.25	$2.60 (2014 prices)

Note: all currency conversions were calculated using the purchasing power parity exchange rate for the year of the original cost estimate. Source: https://data.oecd.org/conversion/purchasing-power-parities-ppp.htm.

In principle, the full spectrum of a screening program or policy also includes the costs of a public health program in coordinating the implementation of screening, reporting of screening results, short and long-term follow-up of screen-positive patients, and the surveillance or tracking of short and long-term outcomes. However, no estimates of public health costs associated with CCHD screening have been published to date.

2.1.1. Labor Cost

The cost of staff time per screen is the product of the average number of minutes per screen and the average wage or labor cost per minute (see Table 2). Empirical screening time estimates can be obtained by either asking nursing staff to estimate their own time or by conducting direct observation, i.e., time-and-motion studies. Three time-and-motion studies conducted in birthing hospitals in three US states using the same data collection methods all calculated that nursing staff took on average 9–10 min per newborn to complete a CCHD screen, including preparation and paperwork [21,23,30]. A similar UK study estimated an average time of 7 min per newborn, but preparation time was minimized because parental consent had been obtained before birth [12]. In contrast, studies based on clinical opinion have assumed that screening takes 2–5 min per newborn [11,13,14,31]. Self-reports by nursing staff in two US hospital-based studies reported average screening times of 3.5–5.5 min per newborn [22,32], although that does not include time spent explaining results to families or documenting screening results [22].

The per-minute cost of staff time for CCHD screening is a function of both the pay scale in a given population and the pay grade of the staff who perform the screening, which can vary by clinical setting and time period. Most programs use registered nurses or midwife staff in a newborn unit. Cost estimates from older studies that used research assistants or physicians to conduct screening do not reflect current hospital procedures. Another source of variability in estimates, at least in US studies, is differences in how labor costs were calculated. Some US studies have considered only hourly wages [22], whereas others included total hourly compensation, including taxes and fringe benefits [21,23]. The most recent UK study cited an official database for unit staff costs [12]. An earlier UK study included an adjustment for administrative overhead as well as benefits [14]. Hourly labor costs differ by occupation and geographic labor market; labor cost per minute was roughly three times higher in a US study conducted in New Jersey [21] than in one conducted in Utah [23] using similar methods (Table 2).

2.1.2. Instruments and Consumables

The equipment cost of CCHD screening consists of the amortized costs of the pulse oximeter machine and reusable probes or sensors and the consumable cost of disposable probes or probe tips and straps. The variety of probe types used for screening creates great heterogeneity in cost estimates. Variable cost per newborn is very low when a reusable probe is used for screening compared to the use of a disposable probe, although there are maintenance costs with reusable probes. A US study conducted by Peterson et al. in a statewide sample of hospitals in New Jersey estimated that the equipment cost per infant screened was $0.49 using fully disposable probes, $1.74 using reusable probes with disposable tips, and $13.62 using disposable probes (2014 USD) [21]. A subsequent US study conducted in two facilities in Utah suggested that the total equipment cost per newborn was $21.92 using disposable probes and $0.25 using reusable probes (2014 USD) [23] (Table 2). British economic evaluations have assumed the use of the less expensive reusable probes [12,14,17].

2.1.3. Diagnostic Work-Up

If a newborn does not pass CCHD screening, the newborn is referred for a diagnostic work-up to determine the cause of hypoxemia, whether cardiac or non-cardiac. The diagnostic process may include a clinical evaluation, laboratory and/or imaging tests (including echocardiography), and possibly transportation to another hospital for further evaluation and management. The diagnostic work-up for non-cardiac causes is variable, and no published studies of CCHD screening to date have included estimates of clinical examination to identify potential non-cardiac causes of hypoxemia. Previous UK studies of CCHD screening costs assumed that newborns who do not pass CCHD screening would receive a 30 min diagnostic echocardiographic assessment by a pediatric cardiologist at a cost of roughly £115 pounds per child (2009 GBP) [12,17]. No cost was assigned in that study for transportation.

Peterson et al. estimated costs of echocardiography based on administrative data from a private insurance claims database, with the analysis restricted to inpatient services during infancy. The cost estimate was a truncated arithmetic mean after excluding the top and bottom 1% of observations [10]. Based on data from Florida, indicating that roughly 43% of infants with CCHD were transferred to another hospital during the birth hospitalization [33], it was assumed that 43% of infants who screened positive would require ambulance transport for transfer to a hospital with echocardiography. The cost of ambulance transport was derived using the same methods as the cost of echocardiography [10]. The additional cost of diagnostic echocardiography and transport was estimated to add $0.25 per newborn screened (2011 USD).

2.1.4. Treatment

The potential reduction in treatment costs associated with timely CCHD diagnosis is challenging to estimate, and only one study to date attempted to do so. In an analysis using linked Florida birth defects surveillance and hospital discharge data from 1998 to 2007, Peterson et al. estimated attributable hospitalization costs in the first year of life for infants with CCHD (n = 3603) [33]. Unadjusted costs were higher for infants with CCHD detected prior to discharge from the birth hospitalization than those detected later because severely affected infants are more likely to be detected sooner and to incur more costly treatment. In a statistical analysis that adjusted for CCHD type, maternal race/ethnicity, and other variables, late CCHD detection was found to be associated with 52% more admissions, 18% more hospitalized days, and 35% higher inpatient costs during infancy relative to the early detection of CCHD [33].

The CEA by Peterson et al. projected the avoided cost of hospitalization for infants with screening-detected CCHD in two steps. First, the difference in number of hospitalized days between infants with timely and late detected CCHD was derived from a previous analysis of Florida data [10,33]. Second, average hospital costs per day among infants with selected CCHD conditions were estimated, assuming that the cost per day was the same for early-detected and late-detected cases [10]. The underlying CEA model assumed that with screening, 77.5% of infants with CCHD would be detected prior to discharge, with an average hospital cost during infancy of $156,501 compared to $181,775 for those not detected, a difference of $24,677 per timely-detected CCHD case (2011 USD). Comparing screening and no-screening scenarios, the hospitalization cost was calculated to be $19,111 per infant with CCHD under screening, taking into account false negatives. That amount was equal to $7.48 per newborn infant (2011 USD) [10].

2.2. Screening Cost per Case Detected

Besides the direct cost of performing screening, it is straightforward to calculate the number of additional cases of CCHD detected in a timely manner due to screening. However, this number must be assessed in a given population, because the numbers of new CCHD diagnoses that can be made through the follow-up of screening using pulse oximetry is dependent on the use and accuracy of prenatal screening and postnatal clinical detection in that population. In particular, an increased frequency of prenatal diagnosis of CCHD results in fewer additional diagnoses of CCHD following CCHD screening using pulse oximetry [34]. The frequency of delayed CCHD diagnoses in the United States was shown to have decreased over time [35], although no decrease in post-discharge CCHD diagnoses was found in a study from the United Kingdom [36].

Multiple studies have estimated the screening cost per CCHD case detected, with widely varying estimates. For example, UK estimates range from roughly £5000 (2001 GBP) [13] to £24,000 (2009 GBP) per CCHD case detected [12] and US estimates range from approximately $21,000 (2011 USD) per case with timely diagnosis [10] to $46,000 (2012 USD) per case detected [22]. Different assumptions about two cost elements—the cost per newborn screened and the averted costs of care resulting from timely diagnosis—account for much of this variation. In particular, some estimates are of gross screening costs and others are net screening costs, after subtracting the avoided cost of treatment. For example, Kochilas et al. reported a relatively high cost per case detected ($46,000), despite assuming a low screening cost [22]. In contrast, Peterson et al. assumed a higher cost of CCHD screening and reported that screening would cost approximately $21,000 per case with timely diagnosis [10]. The Peterson et al. estimate reflected the *net* cost of screening, after subtracting the estimated savings in hospitalization costs during infancy resulting from timely diagnosis, which offset more than half of the screening cost. The gross cost per case detected in that study was roughly $46,000.

As noted in Section 2.1.3, the choice of reusable or disposable pulse oximeter probes can have an even larger impact on estimated costs of CCHD screening. Peterson et al. assumed average equipment and labor costs of $6.86 and $6.62 per infant, respectively (2011 USD) [10]. The equipment cost was derived from a sample of seven New Jersey hospitals, only one of which used fully reusable probes. If it had been assumed that all hospitals used fully reusable probes, the average equipment cost would have been much lower [21], and the average cost per newborn screened would have been roughly half as great.

2.3. Health Gains

It is challenging to estimate health gains from CCHD screening, which encompass avoided early deaths and improved health outcomes among survivors. Cost-effectiveness guidelines call for both types of health outcomes to be expressed in summary measures of health such as the quality-adjusted life-year (QALY) that take into account changes in life expectancy and morbidity [26–28]. However, evidence of improved health among survivors following timely diagnosis is lacking. In addition, it is challenging to find conceptually and empirically appropriate estimates of utility weights for pediatric conditions that can be used to project QALY gains [37–39]. Consequently, it is common for CEAs of interventions that primarily affect survival to calculate the cost per life-year saved, since it makes little practical difference in ranking the cost-effectiveness ratios for such interventions [40].

Two CEA studies published estimates of numbers of deaths avoided through CCHD screening. First, Peterson et al. conservatively assumed that CCHD screening, if applied to four million US births each year, would avoid 20 infant deaths [10]. This estimate was based on a national estimate of 28 annual deaths associated with delayed diagnosis of CCHD in the absence of universal screening. The estimate of 28 deaths was derived by multiplying four million births by an avoidable mortality rate among infants with late-detected CCHD of 1.8% and a frequency of 38.8 infants with late-detected CCHD per 100,000 births, both calculated from a study of linked births and deaths in Florida prior to the introduction of screening [33]; the overall preventable death rate among infants with CCHD was 0.4%. To calculate the number of life-years saved as a denominator for a cost-effectiveness ratio, Peterson et al. took the estimated number of infant deaths averted by screening and multiplied this by 30.7 years, which was the life expectancy at birth of the US population discounted to the present with a 3.0% discount rate per year [10]. In other words, the investigators assumed that surviving infants would have a normal life expectancy.

Tobe et al. estimated infant deaths from CCHD for three scenarios in three Chinese cities [20]. The base scenario assumed that infant mortality would be the same as in the 1950s (standard practice in CEAs is to use recent estimates as the baseline to compare with an intervention). The authors also assumed that "that infant mortality would reduce to approximately 25% if infants received timely diagnosis and treatment", but did not state the assumed mortality rates with and without screening. The ratio of assumed averted deaths to CCHD cases was 0.225 in Beijing, 0.112 in Shandong, and 0.046 in Gansu. They assumed that access to timely diagnosis and treatment varied across regions (e.g., apparently one-half as high in Shandong as in Beijing), but did not make those assumptions explicit. Tobe et al. also reported outcomes in terms of disability-adjusted life-year (DALY) estimates, a measure analogous to the QALY, but did not explain how the DALY estimates were generated [20].

It should be noted that the "disability" weights used to calculate DALYs refer to "any short-term or long-term loss of health" and hence assess morbidity rather than disability [41].

2.4. Cost-Effectiveness Ratios

It is standard practice for CEAs to report incremental cost-effectiveness ratios (ICERs) for interventions that are found to be both more costly (net positive cost) and to improve health outcomes relative to next most cost-effective strategy analyzed. To calculate the numerator of the ICER, analysts are supposed to subtract any cost offset associated with improved health from the cost of the intervention. The denominator is the difference in the number of health outcomes attained, most commonly in the form of discounted life-years or health-adjusted life-years gained relative to the alternative. In some countries, policy makers set threshold values or ranges for ICERs below which interventions are presumed to be considered cost-effective. For example, thresholds for approval of the coverage of new medications have been estimated at roughly £30,000 (GBP) per QALY in the United Kingdom, CAN$50,000 in Canada, and AUS$42,000 in Australia [42].

Peterson et al. projected that the point estimate of the net cost of screening was just over $40,000 per life-year saved in 2011 US dollars [10]. It is increasingly recommended that CEAs include probabilistic sensitivity analyses in which estimates for multiple parameters are allowed to vary simultaneously within ranges using probability distributions and simulation modeling techniques [43]. Peterson et al. also reported that a probabilistic analysis projected a one in three chance that CCHD screening would be cost-saving (i.e., negative net costs), and a roughly four in four probability that CCHD screening would cost less than $100,000 per life-year gained. It should be noted that there is no official threshold or standard for cost-effectiveness in the United States, although a private organization, the Institute for Clinical and Economic Review, has used a range of $100,000 to $150,000 per QALY to establish a "value price" for new therapies [44]. It should also be recognized, though, that because utility weights are usually less than 1.0 and decrease with advancing age, the number of QALYs gained is necessarily less than the number of life-years saved. Consequently, the cost per QALY gained is larger than the cost per life-year gained, often by at least 15–20%, which can affect the interpretation of ICERs relative to benchmark values [24].

CEAs are recommended to report sensitivity analyses that show the dependence of results on uncertainty in estimates or assumptions of model parameters [26–28]. Peterson et al. reported that the three variables with the greatest influence on the cost-effectiveness of CCHD screening were the reduction in hospitalization costs during infancy from early detection, the baseline proportion of late-detected CCHD cases, and the hospital cost of CCHD screening [10]. Variables that had the least influence on the results were the cost of echocardiography, cost and probability of transport for echocardiography and subsequent treatment, the mortality rate among infants with CCHD detected by screening, and the rate of false positives.

It should be noted that the assumption of 18% higher hospitalization costs with the late detection of CCHD assumed a fixed cost per hospital day. However, patients in critical care incur much higher costs per hospital day, and infants with late-detected CCHD are more likely to be in critical care units. The observed difference in hospitalization costs in infancy associated with late detection was twice as large as the difference in hospital days, 35% vs. 18% [33]. Therefore, the CEA was conservative; if the study had assumed 35% lower hospitalization costs in infancy with early detection, the cost-effectiveness ratio could have been close to zero.

Many CEAs reported in low- and middle-income countries use a threshold of three times per capita gross domestic product (GDP) per DALY, which was endorsed in the early 2000s by a World Health Organization report. Using that approach in China, with GDP per capita calculated by province, Tobe et al. concluded, "the intervention was highly cost-effective in Beijing (Int$7833/DALY); cost-effective in Shandong (Int$27,780/DALY); and not cost-effective in Gansu (Int$167,407)" [20]. However, those are average cost-effectiveness ratios rather than ICERs. The authors' Table 1 indicates ICERs for CCHD screening of Int$15,020, Int$51,636, and Int$307,952, respectively. If the same arbitrary cost-effectiveness threshold had been applied to the ICERs, CCHD screening would not have been considered cost-effective in either Shandong or Gansu. In addition, it should be noted that the three times GDP per capita cost-effectiveness threshold value has been challenged as lacking validity [45].

3. Revised Cost-Effectiveness Estimates

3.1. New Estimates of Averted Infant Deaths

Newly published estimates of the impact of CCHD screening policies in the United States suggest that the actual reduction in CCHD deaths associated with universal screening may be much higher than previous economic evaluations anticipated. A statistical analysis of the association of US state CCHD screening policies that had been adopted by 1 June 2013 with the numbers of early infant (24 h to <6 months of age) deaths coded for CCHD or other/unspecified congenital heart defects (CHDs) through the end of 2013 found that the implementation of CCHD screening mandates was associated with a one-third lower frequency of recognized infant deaths with CCHD as the listed cause (see Supplement) [46]. The reduction in CCHD deaths was not entirely attributable to screening using pulse oximetry, since screening mandates could also have led to a greater clinical awareness and the earlier detection of CCHD using other methods. This reduction in CCHD-associated deaths was roughly six times greater than was assumed in the US CEA of CCHD screening by Peterson et al. based on the frequency of delayed CCHD diagnoses that could be avoided through screening [10]. Adjusting the Peterson et al. model to include 110 deaths averted annually (as opposed to the 20 deaths averted annually assumed in the Peterson et al. original study), the estimated cost per life-year gained becomes approximately $10,000 (2011 USD) (compared to the original reported estimate of approximately $40,000 per life-year gained).

3.2. Shortened Life Expectancy among Survivors

One factor unaddressed by Peterson et al. and other economic evaluations of CCHD screening is shortened life expectancy among individuals with CCHD. In other words, previous economic evaluations have implicitly or explicitly assumed that children with CCHD who survive infancy have the same life expectancy as unaffected children. However, all-cause mortality is higher among children with CHDs than for the general population, even after infancy [47]. For example, it has been widely reported that children and adolescents with CHDs have higher rates of cancer, even after excluding individuals with chromosomal disorders [48]. Survival with a CHD varies widely by condition or type of defect, country, ethnic group, and time period. Dramatic reductions over time in infant and early childhood mortality among cohorts of infants born with a CHD have been widely reported [49–52].

Few studies have reported survival probabilities for patients with CHDs relative to life-table survival probabilities for the general population. A population-based surveillance study conducted in metropolitan Atlanta, Georgia (USA), involving birth cohorts from 1979 to 2005, found that the average infant survival probability for infants with CCHD who had no non-cardiac defects or chromosomal syndromes was 75.2%, but increased from 67.2% during the first 15 years to 82.5% during the more recent 12 years [52]. One implication of the reductions in infant deaths associated with CCHD is a smaller number of deaths that could be potentially averted through screening. The average survival probability from 12 months to 25 years of age was 89.3%, which compares with a 99.3% survival probability for the general US population in the 2009 national life table [53]. A Danish study modeled post-surgery survival to age 25 among children born during 1990–2002 as 85% for all CHDs and from 64% to 87% for specific CCHD types, but the 10-year survival probability for the subsequent birth cohort was substantially greater, 93% vs. 87% overall [54].

It would be reasonable to project that life expectancy among individuals with CCHD who survive infancy could be 10–20% lower than in the general population. That would reduce discounted life-years by three to six years relative to population norms. Adjusting the US CEA model of CCHD screening reported by Peterson et al. to include 110 deaths averted annually and 20% fewer years lived yields an estimated cost per life-year saved of approximately $12,000 (2011 USD).

3.3. CHD-Related Future Medical Costs

It is generally recommended that CEAs include the present value of expected future medical costs for survivors whose deaths are avoided or postponed as a result of a healthcare intervention, although only one-half of CEAs published during 2008–2013 included estimates of future related medical costs [55]. Since infants with complex medical conditions incur substantial medical costs, including future medical costs can make life-saving interventions for such children appear less cost-effective. It is common for CEAs of newborn screening tests to not include future medical costs [40].

No estimates of lifetime medical costs for children with CHDs in general or for the subset with CCHD defects are currently available, with or without adjustment for co-occurring conditions. A US study that used linked birth defects surveillance and administrative data from California dating from the late 1980s estimated lifetime costs for four infants born with one of four specific CCHD conditions: truncus arteriosus, transposition of the great arteries/double-outlet right ventricle, tetralogy of Fallot, and single ventricle [56]. At the time of the study, infant survival was assumed to be low, with <50% of infants with truncus arteriosus or single ventricle reaching one year of age. A CDC publication recalculated the cost estimates with a 3% discount rate; lifetime medical costs per infant varied by condition from $86,000 to $260,000 (1992 USD) [57].

Given dramatic changes in survival and medical technologies, cost estimates from three decades in the past are not currently informative [58]. An analysis of 2005 US private insurance claims data reported that children with severe CHDs (roughly equivalent to CCHD) had mean expenditures during the first three years of life of roughly $210,000 in excess of children without CHDs [58]. The most recent estimates of hospitalization costs associated with birth defects estimated an aggregate burden almost twice as high in 2013 as in 2004 [59]. In 2013, the mean cost for a single inpatient stay with a CCHD diagnosis was $79,011, and aggregate hospital costs for CCHD patients of all ages generated a figure of $2.3 billion [59].

Despite the absence of recent estimates of lifetime costs for infants born with CCHD, it is possible to conduct sensitivity analyses. One potential proxy is the lifetime medical cost for infants born with spina bifida, which was recently estimated as $513,500 (2014 USD) [60]. In the analysis of California data from the late 1980s, medical costs for children born with spina bifida were similar to those born with single ventricle or tetralogy of Fallot and lower than those with truncus arteriosus [56,57]. However, annual medical costs for spina bifida remain elevated across the lifespan [60], whereas costs associated with care for severe CHDs drop off sharply after infancy. Roughly two-thirds of all hospital costs associated with CHD diagnoses are associated with admissions in the first 12 months of life [61]. Therefore, the lifetime medical cost for spina bifida might be an upper-bound estimate of the lifetime medical cost associated with CCHD.

Adjusting the US CEA model of CCHD screening reported by Peterson et al. to include 110 deaths averted annually, 20% fewer years lived, and $450,000 in post-infancy CCHD-attributable discounted future lifetime medical costs (as opposed to $0 included in the original study), yields an estimated cost per life-year saved of approximately $31,000 (2011 USD). That sensitivity analysis yields a conservative estimate of net benefit (i.e., the cost-effectiveness ratio is likely overestimated) since the actual incremental medical cost associated with CCHD is likely less than the proxy estimate that was used. In any case, the estimated cost is still lower than the originally reported estimate of approximately $40,000 per life-year gained.

4. Discussion

To date, all economic analyses of CCHD screening have followed the healthcare sector perspective, as is conventional for clinical interventions. All have included employee compensation costs to employers to estimate the cost of staff time. However, hospitals that have implemented CCHD screening have reported to be able to do so using existing nursing staff and do not incur additional staff costs [21]. From the hospital perspective, the cost of staff time might not need to be included [10]. From a societal perspective, the inclusion of staff time makes sense if nursing time used for CCHD screening could have otherwise been used for other tasks. If nursing time could not be reallocated, the time spent doing the screening would not represent an incremental cost. If that is the case, existing cost estimates could overestimate the incremental cost of CCHD screening.

Economic analyses of CCHD screening as a public policy should also include the costs of public health activities in support of CCHD screening and follow-up, but little is known about those costs. Jurisdictions implementing CCHD screening policies and programs often take varying approaches to the organization and surveillance of CCHD screening [62]. For that reason, it may not be possible to generalize the costs of the public health role in supporting and monitoring CCHD screening.

Notable variations exist in methods and results among the two previously published CEAs of CCHD screening [10,20] and several costing studies included in this review. The level of evidence for some cost elements, notably the cost of CCHD screening based on combined screening time, labor cost, instrumentation, and consumables cost, is reasonably established in some clinical settings. These cost elements still merit reconsideration or reinvestigation for future economic evaluations, for each is dependent on existing conditions in a given clinical setting. Estimates of effectiveness are also variable. Survival among infants with CCHD can vary greatly depending on location and treatment availability, which limits the generalizability of results across settings within countries, as well as across countries.

Other formal healthcare costs associated with CCHD screening are less well established. Some matter more than others, as indicated by their potential magnitude per infant screened. For example, the cost of the diagnostic work-up of screen-positive newborns is not well established, but given the very small numbers of infants who screen positive, this cost element contributes very little to the total cost of screening; perhaps 2% of the total cost [10]. It is likely that the assumption in the Peterson et al. study that 43% of newborns who do not pass CCHD screening require transport to another hospital is a substantial overestimate, but since such transportation contributed only marginally to the estimated total cost of screening in that study, modifying that assumption would have little effect on the results. In contrast, the cost of avoided hospitalizations associated with late-detected CCHD is highly influential [10]. However, that cost estimate in Peterson et al. was based on just one study in one US state conducted prior to the implementation of universal CCHD screening [33]. Furthermore, the Peterson et al. study assumed a high rate of sensitivity of CCHD screening.

Some healthcare costs have been neglected in economic evaluations of CCHD screening. One is the cost and benefits of diagnosing and treating non-CCHD cases among newborns referred following screening. The implicit assumption has been that the costs of diagnostic work-up relative to the size of the newborn population are low, similar to that of CCHD diagnosis. However, the potential health benefits of detecting and treating non-cardiac conditions, such as neonatal sepsis, deserve further attention. Non-health costs have been neglected in published cost-effectiveness analyses of CCHD screening to date. For example, no published information exists on the time costs incurred by family members caring for individuals with CCHD, nor the loss of economic productivity. Although there is evidence of the increased use of special education services among surviving children with CCHD [63,64], the associated costs have not been calculated. Furthermore, it is unknown whether early detection might influence long-term academic outcomes among those children.

Three parameters can substantially affect the overall CEA results and remain underinvestigated: estimates of averted infant CCHD deaths, shortened life expectancy among children with CCHD who survive infancy, and future CCHD-associated medical costs. Previous CEAs have relied on indirect estimates of averted deaths based on estimates of numbers of infant deaths with CCHD, the frequency of delayed diagnosis, and the assumed relative reduction with timely diagnosis; they have excluded the other two parameters. For example, Peterson et al. calculated an expected number of averted deaths based on infant mortality differentials by timing of diagnosis derived before the advent of universal screening [10]. Newly available estimates of the relative reduction in deaths associated with CCHD screening mandates based on a retrospective analysis of CCHD deaths in US states with universal screening policies offer evidence of a greater number of deaths averted [46] than had been projected by Peterson et al. [10] Using the direct estimates of averted deaths associated with mandatory CCHD screening policies from Abouk et al. [46] yields cost-effectiveness ratios more favorable for universal screening policies.

A comparative analysis of life expectancy among CCHD survivors relative to the general population can contribute evidence to improve future economic evaluations of CCHD screening. Where previous CEAs have assumed a normal life expectancy for individuals that through CCHD screening detection avoided CCHD-associated death, accounting for a shorter than average life expectancy will increase the net cost of screening by increasing the cost per life-year gained. Finally, previous CEAs have not accounted for CCHD-related expenditures associated with averted CCHD death in infancy. Accounting for such costs will also presumably increase the net cost of CCHD screening.

In conclusion, uncertainty remains regarding several parameters that are important to the analysis of the cost-effectiveness of CCHD screening. Nonetheless, the ability of universal CCHD screening to detect many newborns with CCHD who would otherwise have remained undiagnosed at the time of discharge—and at risk of severe morbidity and mortality—has been demonstrated [65–67].

Supplementary Materials: The following are available online at www.mdpi.com/2409-515X/3/4/34/s1. References [46,68] are cited in the supplementary materials.

Acknowledgments: No funding was received for the preparation or publication of the study.

Disclaimer: The findings and conclusions in this report are those of the authors and do not necessarily represent the official position of the Centers for Disease Control and Prevention.

Author Contributions: Scott D. Grosse and Cora Peterson conceived the review and the new, updated results. Scott D. Grosse conducted the review and wrote most of the paper. Rahi Abouk produced the new estimates of avoided deaths and contributed to the new cost-effectiveness estimates. Jill Glidewell and Matthew E. Oster provided substantive input and clinical expertise in the interpretation of the findings. All authors contributed to the final version of the paper.

Conflicts of Interest: The authors declare no conflict of interest.

References

1. Centers for Disease Control and Prevention. CDC Grand Rounds: Newborn screening and improved outcomes. *Morb. Mortal. Wkly. Rep.* **2012**, *61*, 390–393.
2. Wilson, J.M.; Jungner, Y.G. Principles and practice of mass screening for disease. *Bol. Oficina Sanit. Panam.* **1968**, *65*, 281–393. [PubMed]
3. Grosse, S.D.; Thompson, J.D.; Ding, Y.; Glass, M. The use of economic evaluation to inform newborn screening policy decisions: The Washington state experience. *Milbank Q.* **2016**, *94*, 366–391. [CrossRef] [PubMed]
4. Fischer, K.E.; Grosse, S.D.; Rogowski, W.H. The role of health technology assessment in coverage decisions on newborn screening. *Int. J. Technol. Assess. Health Care* **2011**, *27*, 313–321. [CrossRef] [PubMed]
5. Grosse, S.D. Cost effectiveness as a criterion for newborn screening policy decisions. In *Ethics and Newborn Genetic Screening: New Technologies, New Challenges*; Baily, M.A., Murray, T.H., Eds.; Johns Hopkins University Press: Baltimore, MD, USA, 2009; pp. 58–88.
6. Grosse, S.D.; Riehle-Colarusso, T.; Gaffney, M.; Mason, C.A.; Shapira, S.K.; Sontag, M.K.; Braun, K.V.N.; Iskander, J. CDC Grand Rounds: Newborn screening for hearing loss and critical congenital heart disease. *Morb. Mortal. Wkly. Rep.* **2017**, *66*, 888–890. [CrossRef] [PubMed]
7. Ewer, A.K. Review of pulse oximetry screening for critical congenital heart defects in newborn infants. *Curr. Opin. Cardiol.* **2013**, *28*, 92–96. [CrossRef] [PubMed]
8. Sebelius, K. Letter to the Secretary's Advisory Council on Hereditary Diseases of Newborns and Children. Available online: http://www.hrsa.gov/advisorycommittees/mchbadvisory/heritabledisorders/recommendations/correspondence/cyanoticheartsecre09212011.pdf (accessed on 20 July 2016).

9. Martin, G.R.; Beekman, R.H., III; Mikula, E.B.; Fasules, J.; Garg, L.F.; Kemper, A.R.; Morrow, W.R.; Pearson, G.D.; Mahle, W.T. Implementing recommended screening for critical congenital heart disease. *Pediatrics* **2013**, *132*, e185–e192. [CrossRef] [PubMed]
10. Peterson, C.; Grosse, S.D.; Oster, M.E.; Olney, R.S.; Cassell, C.H. Cost-effectiveness of routine screening for critical congenital heart disease in US newborns. *Pediatrics* **2013**, *132*, e595–e603. [CrossRef] [PubMed]
11. De-Wahl Granelli, A.; Wennergren, M.; Sandberg, K.; Mellander, M.; Bejlum, C.; Inganas, L.; Eriksson, M.; Segerdahl, N.; Agren, A.; Ekman-Joelsson, B.M.; et al. Impact of pulse oximetry screening on the detection of duct dependent congenital heart disease: A Swedish prospective screening study in 39,821 newborns. *BMJ* **2009**, *338*, a3037. [CrossRef] [PubMed]
12. Roberts, T.E.; Barton, P.M.; Auguste, P.E.; Middleton, L.J.; Furmston, A.T.; Ewer, A.K. Pulse oximetry as a screening test for congenital heart defects in newborn infants: A cost-effectiveness analysis. *Arch. Dis. Child.* **2012**, *97*, 221–226. [CrossRef] [PubMed]
13. Griebsch, I.; Knowles, R.L.; Brown, J.; Bull, C.; Wren, C.; Dezateux, C.A. Comparing the clinical and economic effects of clinical examination, pulse oximetry, and echocardiography in newborn screening for congenital heart defects: A probabilistic cost-effectiveness model and value of information analysis. *Int. J. Technol. Assess. Health Care* **2007**, *23*, 192–204. [CrossRef] [PubMed]
14. Knowles, R.; Griebsch, I.; Dezateux, C.; Brown, J.; Bull, C.; Wren, C. Newborn screening for congenital heart defects: A systematic review and cost-effectiveness analysis. *Health Technol. Assess.* **2005**, *9*, 1–152. [CrossRef] [PubMed]
15. Ewer, A.K.; Furmston, A.T.; Middleton, L.J.; Deeks, J.J.; Daniels, J.P.; Pattison, H.M.; Powell, R.; Roberts, T.E.; Barton, P.; Auguste, P.; et al. Pulse oximetry as a screening test for congenital heart defects in newborn infants: A test accuracy study with evaluation of acceptability and cost-effectiveness. *Health Technol. Assess.* **2012**, *16*, 1–184. [CrossRef] [PubMed]
16. Mahle, W.T.; Newburger, J.W.; Matherne, G.P.; Smith, F.C.; Hoke, T.R.; Koppel, R.; Gidding, S.S.; Beekman, R.H., III; Grosse, S.D. Role of pulse oximetry in examining newborns for congenital heart disease: A scientific statement from the American Heart Association and American Academy of Pediatrics. *Circulation* **2009**, *120*, 447–458. [CrossRef] [PubMed]
17. Ewer, A.K.; Middleton, L.J.; Furmston, A.T.; Bhoyar, A.; Daniels, J.P.; Thangaratinam, S.; Deeks, J.J.; Khan, K.S.; PulseOx Study Group. Pulse oximetry screening for congenital heart defects in newborn infants (PulseOx): A test accuracy study. *Lancet* **2011**, *378*, 785–794. [CrossRef]
18. Grosse, S.D. Showing value in newborn screening: Challenges in quantifying the effectiveness and cost-effectiveness of early detection of phenylketonuria and cystic fibrosis. *Healthcare* **2015**, *3*, 1133–1157. [CrossRef] [PubMed]
19. Grosse, S.D. Assessing cost-effectiveness in healthcare: History of the $50,000 per QALY threshold. *Expert Rev. Pharmacoecon. Outcomes Res.* **2008**, *8*, 165–178. [CrossRef] [PubMed]
20. Tobe, R.G.; Martin, G.R.; Li, F.; Mori, R. Should postnatal oximetry screening be implemented nationwide in China? A cost-effectiveness analysis in three regions with different socioeconomic status. *Int. J. Cardiol.* **2016**, *204*, 45–47. [CrossRef] [PubMed]
21. Peterson, C.; Grosse, S.D.; Glidewell, J.; Garg, L.F.; Van Naarden Braun, K.; Knapp, M.M.; Beres, L.M.; Hinton, C.F.; Olney, R.S.; Cassell, C.H. A public health economic assessment of hospitals' cost to screen newborns for critical congenital heart disease. *Public Health Rep.* **2014**, *129*, 86–93. [CrossRef] [PubMed]
22. Kochilas, L.K.; Lohr, J.L.; Bruhn, E.; Borman-Shoap, E.; Gams, B.L.; Pylipow, M.; Saarinen, A.; Gaviglio, A.; Thompson, T.R. Implementation of critical congenital heart disease screening in Minnesota. *Pediatrics* **2013**, *132*, e587–e594. [CrossRef] [PubMed]
23. Reeder, M.R.; Kim, J.; Nance, A.; Krikov, S.; Feldkamp, M.L.; Randall, H.; Botto, L.D. Evaluating cost and resource use associated with pulse oximetry screening for critical congenital heart disease: Empiric estimates and sources of variation. *Birth Defects Res. A Clin. Mol. Teratol.* **2015**, *103*, 962–971. [CrossRef] [PubMed]
24. Grosse, S.D. When is genomic testing cost-effective? Testing for Lynch Syndrome in patients with newly-diagnosed colorectal cancer and their relatives. *Healthcare* **2015**, *3*, 860–878. [CrossRef] [PubMed]
25. Hatz, M.H.; Schremser, K.; Rogowski, W.H. Is individualized medicine more cost-effective? A systematic review. *Pharmacoeconomics* **2014**, *32*, 443–455. [CrossRef] [PubMed]
26. Drummond, M.E.; O'Brien, B.; Stoddart, G.L.; Torrance, G.W. *Methods for the Economic Evaluation of Health Care Programmes*, 2nd ed.; Oxford University Press: Oxford, UK, 1997.

27. Gold, M.R.; Siegel, J.E.; Russell, L.B.; Weinstein, M.C. *Cost-Effectiveness in Health and Medicine*; Oxford University Press: New York, NY, USA, 1996.
28. Sanders, G.D.; Neumann, P.J.; Basu, A.; Brock, D.W.; Feeny, D.; Krahn, M.; Kuntz, K.M.; Meltzer, D.O.; Owens, D.K.; Prosser, L.A.; et al. Recommendations for conduct, methodological practices, and reporting of cost-effectiveness analyses: Second Panel on Cost-Effectiveness in Health and Medicine. *JAMA* **2016**, *316*, 1093–1103. [CrossRef] [PubMed]
29. Tilford, J.M.; Payakachat, N. Progress in measuring family spillover effects for economic evaluations. *Expert Rev. Pharmacoecon. Outcomes Res.* **2015**, *15*, 195–198. [CrossRef] [PubMed]
30. Centers for Disease Control and Prevention. Assessment of current practices and feasibility of routine screening for critical congenital heart defects—Georgia, 2012. *Morb. Mortal. Wkly. Rep.* **2013**, *62*, 288–291.
31. Walsh, W. Evaluation of pulse oximetry screening in Middle Tennessee: Cases for consideration before universal screening. *J. Perinatol.* **2011**, *31*, 125–129. [CrossRef] [PubMed]
32. Bradshaw, E.A.; Cuzzi, S.; Kiernan, S.C.; Nagel, N.; Becker, J.A.; Martin, G.R. Feasibility of implementing pulse oximetry screening for congenital heart disease in a community hospital. *J. Perinatol.* **2012**, *32*, 710–715. [CrossRef] [PubMed]
33. Peterson, C.; Dawson, A.; Grosse, S.D.; Riehle-Colarusso, T.; Olney, R.S.; Tanner, J.P.; Kirby, R.S.; Correia, J.A.; Watkins, S.M.; Cassell, C.H. Hospitalizations, costs, and mortality among infants with critical congenital heart disease: How important is timely detection? *Birth Defects Res. A Clin. Mol. Teratol.* **2013**, *97*, 664–672. [CrossRef] [PubMed]
34. Ailes, E.C.; Gilboa, S.M.; Honein, M.A.; Oster, M.E. Estimated number of infants detected and missed by critical congenital heart defect screening. *Pediatrics* **2015**, *135*, 1000–1008. [CrossRef] [PubMed]
35. Chang, R.K.; Gurvitz, M.; Rodriguez, S. Missed diagnosis of critical congenital heart disease. *Arch. Pediatr. Adolesc. Med.* **2008**, *162*, 969–974. [CrossRef] [PubMed]
36. Wren, C.; Reinhardt, Z.; Khawaja, K. Twenty-year trends in diagnosis of life-threatening neonatal cardiovascular malformations. *Arch Dis. Child. Fetal Neonatal Ed.* **2008**, *93*, F33–F35. [CrossRef] [PubMed]
37. Grosse, S.D.; Prosser, L.A.; Asakawa, K.; Feeny, D. QALY weights for neurosensory impairments in pediatric economic evaluations: Case studies and a critique. *Expert Rev. Pharmacoecon. Outcomes Res.* **2010**, *10*, 293–308. [CrossRef] [PubMed]
38. Ungar, W.J. Challenges in health state valuation in paediatric economic evaluation: Are QALYs contraindicated? *Pharmacoeconomics* **2011**, *29*, 641–652. [CrossRef] [PubMed]
39. Grosse, S.D. Economic evaluations of newborn screening interventions. In *Economic Evaluation in Child Health*; Ungar, W.J., Ed.; Oxford University Press: New York, NY, USA, 2009; pp. 113–132.
40. Ding, Y.; Thompson, J.D.; Kobrynski, L.; Ojodu, J.; Zarbalian, G.; Grosse, S.D. Cost-Effectiveness/Cost-Benefit Analysis of Newborn Screening for Severe Combined Immune Deficiency in Washington State. *J. Pediatr.* **2016**, *172*, 127–135. [CrossRef] [PubMed]
41. Salomon, J.A.; Vos, T.; Hogan, D.R.; Gagnon, M.; Naghavi, M.; Mokdad, A.; Begum, N.; Shah, R.; Karyana, M.; Kosen, S.; et al. Common values in assessing health outcomes from disease and injury: Disability weights measurement study for the Global Burden of Disease Study 2010. *Lancet* **2012**, *380*, 2129–2143. [CrossRef]
42. Griffiths, E.A.; Hendrich, J.K.; Stoddart, S.D.; Walsh, S.C. Acceptance of health technology assessment submissions with incremental cost-effectiveness ratios above the cost-effectiveness threshold. *Clinicoecon. Outcomes Res.* **2015**, *7*, 463–476. [CrossRef] [PubMed]
43. Briggs, A.H.; Weinstein, M.C.; Fenwick, E.A.; Karnon, J.; Sculpher, M.J.; Paltiel, A.D.; Ispor-Smdm Modeling Good Research Practices Task Force. Model parameter estimation and uncertainty analysis: A report of the ISPOR-SMDM Modeling Good Research Practices Task Force Working Group-6. *Med. Decis. Mak.* **2012**, *32*, 722–732. [CrossRef] [PubMed]
44. Neumann, P.J.; Cohen, J.T. ICER's revised value assessment framework for 2017-2019: A critique. *Pharmacoeconomics* **2017**, *35*, 977–980. [CrossRef] [PubMed]
45. Marseille, E.; Larson, B.; Kazi, D.S.; Kahn, J.G.; Rosen, S. Thresholds for the cost-effectiveness of interventions: Alternative approaches. *Bull. World Health Organ.* **2015**, *93*, 118–124. [CrossRef] [PubMed]
46. Abouk, R.; Grosse, S.D.; Ailes, E.C.; Oster, M.E. Association of US state implementation of newborn screening policies for critical congenital heart disease with early infant cardiac deaths. *JAMA* **2017**, *318*, 2111–2118. [CrossRef] [PubMed]

47. Best, K.E.; Rankin, J. Long-term survival of individuals born with congenital heart disease: A systematic review and meta-analysis. *J. Am. Heart Assoc.* **2016**, *5*, e002846. [CrossRef] [PubMed]
48. Botto, L.D.; Flood, T.; Little, J.; Fluchel, M.N.; Krikov, S.; Feldkamp, M.L.; Wu, Y.; Goedken, R.; Puzhankara, S.; Romitti, P.A. Cancer risk in children and adolescents with birth defects: A population-based cohort study. *PLoS ONE* **2013**, *8*, e69077. [CrossRef] [PubMed]
49. Khairy, P.; Ionescu-Ittu, R.; Mackie, A.S.; Abrahamowicz, M.; Pilote, L.; Marelli, A.J. Changing mortality in congenital heart disease. *J. Am. Coll. Cardiol.* **2010**, *56*, 1149–1157. [CrossRef] [PubMed]
50. Nembhard, W.N.; Salemi, J.L.; Ethen, M.K.; Fixler, D.E.; Dimaggio, A.; Canfield, M.A. Racial/Ethnic disparities in risk of early childhood mortality among children with congenital heart defects. *Pediatrics* **2011**, *127*, e1128–e1138. [CrossRef] [PubMed]
51. Wang, Y.; Liu, G.; Druschel, C.M.; Kirby, R.S. Maternal race/ethnicity and survival experience of children with congenital heart disease. *J. Pediatr.* **2013**, *163*, 1437–1442. [CrossRef] [PubMed]
52. Oster, M.E.; Lee, K.A.; Honein, M.A.; Riehle-Colarusso, T.; Shin, M.; Correa, A. Temporal trends in survival among infants with critical congenital heart defects. *Pediatrics* **2013**, *131*, e1502–e1508. [CrossRef] [PubMed]
53. Arias, E. United States Life Tables, 2009. In *National Vital Statistics Reports*; Centers for Disease Control and Prevention, National Center for Health Statistics, National Vital Statistics System: Atlanta, GA, USA, 2014; Volume 62, pp. 1–63.
54. Larsen, S.H.; Olsen, M.; Emmertsen, K.; Hjortdal, V.E. Interventional treatment of patients with congenital heart disease: Nationwide Danish experience over 39 years. *J. Am. Coll. Cardiol.* **2017**, *69*, 2725–2732. [CrossRef] [PubMed]
55. Gros, B.; Soto Alvarez, J.; Angel Casado, M. Incorporation of future costs in health economic analysis publications: Current situation and recommendations for the future. *Expert Rev. Pharmacoecon. Outcomes Res.* **2015**, *15*, 465–469. [CrossRef] [PubMed]
56. Waitzman, N.J.; Romano, P.S.; Scheffler, R.M. *The Cost of Birth Defects*; University Press of America: Lanham, MD, USA, 1996.
57. Centers for Disease Control and Prevention. Economic costs of birth defects and cerebral palsy—United States, 1992. *Morb. Mortal. Wkly. Rep.* **1995**, *44*, 694–699.
58. Boulet, S.; Grosse, S.; Riehle-Colarusso, T.; Correa-Villasenor, A. Health care costs of congenital heart defects. In *Congenital Heart Defects: From Origin to Treatment*; Wyszynski, D., Graham, T., Correa-Villasenor, A., Eds.; Oxford University Press: New York, NY, USA, 2010; pp. 493–501.
59. Arth, A.C.; Tinker, S.C.; Simeone, R.M.; Ailes, E.C.; Cragan, J.D.; Grosse, S.D. Inpatient hospitalization costs associated with birth defects among persons of all ages—United States, 2013. *Morb. Mortal. Wkly. Rep.* **2017**, *66*, 41–46. [CrossRef] [PubMed]
60. Grosse, S.D.; Berry, R.J.; Tilford, J.M.; Kucik, J.E.; Waitzman, N.J. Retrospective assessment of cost savings from prevention: Folic acid fortification and spina bifida in the US. *Am. J. Prev. Med.* **2016**, *50*, S74–S80. [CrossRef] [PubMed]
61. Simeone, R.M.; Oster, M.E.; Hobbs, C.A.; Robbins, J.M.; Collins, R.T.; Honein, M.A. Population-based study of hospital costs for hospitalizations of infants, children, and adults with a congenital heart defect, Arkansas 2006 to 2011. *Birth Defects Res. A Clin. Mol. Teratol.* **2015**, *103*, 814–820. [CrossRef] [PubMed]
62. Glidewell, J.; Olney, R.S.; Hinton, C.; Pawelski, J.; Sontag, M.; Wood, T.; Kucik, J.E.; Daskalov, R.; Hudson, J. State legislation, regulations, and hospital guidelines for newborn screening for critical congenital heart defects—United States, 2011–2014. *Morb. Mortal. Wkly. Rep.* **2015**, *64*, 625–630.
63. Oster, M.E.; Watkins, S.; Hill, K.D.; Knight, J.H.; Meyer, R.E. Academic outcomes in children with congenital heart defects: A population-based cohort study. *Circ. Cardiovasc. Qual. Outcomes* **2017**, *10*, e003074. [CrossRef] [PubMed]
64. Riehle-Colarusso, T.; Autry, A.; Razzaghi, H.; Boyle, C.A.; Mahle, W.T.; Van Naarden Braun, K.; Correa, A. Congenital heart defects and receipt of special education services. *Pediatrics* **2015**, *136*, 496–504. [CrossRef] [PubMed]
65. Ismail, A.Q.; Cawsey, M.; Ewer, A.K. Newborn pulse oximetry screening in practice. *Arch. Dis. Child. Educ. Pract. Ed.* **2016**, *102*, 155–161. [CrossRef] [PubMed]
66. Oster, M.E.; Aucott, S.W.; Glidewell, J.; Hackell, J.; Kochilas, L.; Martin, G.R.; Phillippi, J.; Pinto, N.M.; Saarinen, A.; Sontag, M.; et al. Lessons learned from newborn screening for critical congenital heart defects. *Pediatrics* **2016**, *137*, e20154573. [CrossRef] [PubMed]

67. Narayen, I.C.; Blom, N.A.; Ewer, A.K.; Vento, M.; Manzoni, P.; te Pas, A.B. Aspects of pulse oximetry screening for critical congenital heart defects: When, how and why? *Arch. Dis. Child. Fetal Neonatal Ed.* **2016**, *101*, F162–F167. [CrossRef] [PubMed]
68. Martin, J.A.; Hamilton, B.E.; Osterman, M.J. Births in the United States, 2015. *NCHS Data Brief* **2016**, 1–8.

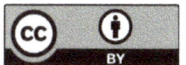

© 2017 by the authors. Licensee MDPI, Basel, Switzerland. This article is an open access article distributed under the terms and conditions of the Creative Commons Attribution (CC BY) license (http://creativecommons.org/licenses/by/4.0/).

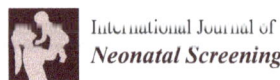

Review

Barriers to the Implementation of Newborn Pulse Oximetry Screening: A Different Perspective

Martin Kluckow

Department of Neonatal Medicine, Royal North Shore Hospital and University of Sydney, Sydney, NSW 2065, Australia; martin.kluckow@sydney.edu.au; Tel.: +61-2-9463-2180

Received: 8 November 2017; Accepted: 8 January 2018; Published: 11 January 2018

Abstract: Pulse oximetry screening of the well newborn to assist in the diagnosis of critical congenital heart disease (CCHD) is increasingly being adopted. There are advantages to diagnosing CCHD prior to collapse, particularly if this occurs outside of the hospital setting. The current recommended approach links pulse oximetry screening with the assessment for CCHD. An alternative approach is to document the oxygen saturation as part of a routine set of vital signs in each newborn infant prior to discharge, delinking the measurement of oxygen saturation from assessment for CCHD. This approach, the way that many hospitals which contribute to the Australian New Zealand Neonatal Network (ANZNN) have introduced screening, has the potential benefits of decreasing parental anxiety and expectation, not requiring specific consent, changing the interpretation of false positives and therefore the timing of the test, and removing the pressure to perform an immediate echocardiogram if the test is positive. There are advantages of introducing a formal screening program, including the attainment of adequate funding and a universal approach, but the barriers noted above need to be dealt with and the process of acceptance by a national body as a screening test can take many years.

Keywords: pulse oximetry; neonate; congenital heart disease; screening

1. Introduction

Reviews suggest that about 30% of infants with critical congenital heart disease (CCHD) leave hospital undiagnosed and that, in cardiovascular deaths occurring within the first week of life, the malformation was not identified before death in one out of four [1,2]. Neurological outcome is related to the presentation of the disease, with infants who collapse prior to presentation having a significantly worse outcome than those that are identified prior to collapse [3]. There is therefore a need for the development of effective screening tests for CCHD. Current screening for congenital heart defects has relied on a mid-trimester ultrasound scan, which is operator-dependent and at present detects <50% of CHD and about 60% of CCHD requiring surgery in the first month of life [4,5]. In Sweden, 26% of newborns with CCHD were sent home without being diagnosed [6].

Pulse oximetry has been evaluated in multiple studies as a screening test for CCHD. A high sensitivity is clearly important where a test is used to screen for a serious but treatable disease. Ewer et al. [7] in a test accuracy study showed that pulse oximetry had a sensitivity of 58% for critical (likely to require treatment in the first month) and 29% for all major (likely to require treatment in the first year) lesions when antenatal screening was negative. A systematic review and meta-analysis by Thangaratinam et al. [8] including 13 studies and almost 230,000 babies showed the overall sensitivity of pulse oximetry for the detection of critical congenital heart defects was 76.5%. In this review, there were no significant differences in sensitivity for pulse oximetry in the foot alone versus in both foot and right hand. The specificity was 99.9%, with an overall false-positive rate of 0.14%. The equipment is readily available and does not require calibration; the monitoring is minimally invasive and familiar to most parents and staff. Despite all of these potential screening advantages, the uptake of pulse oximetry screening for CCHD has not been universal. This paper aims to identify and review the barriers to the implementation of pulse oximetry as a screening test for CCHD.

2. Australian/New Zealand Progress

The adoption of pulse oximetry for screening for critical congenital heart disease has progressed substantially around the world, led by the development and adoption of screening guidelines in North America by the American Academy of Pediatrics (AAP) in 2011 [9]. The adoption of pulse oximetry screening in Australia/New Zealand has been on a hospital-by-hospital, state-by-state basis. New Zealand has recently proposed a countrywide adoption of screening at all health care facility levels and is currently exploring the feasibility of this [10]. A recent survey of all of the Australian/New Zealand Neonatal Intensive Care Units (Unpublished 2017) concluded that 77% of all units have implemented a screening program. Three units in New Zealand were not screening pending the introduction of a National screening program. Two units in Australia had suspended their screening programs due to resourcing implications both at the primary screen and in dealing with positive test results. Most units have adopted a screening guideline similar to either the AAP-recommended one or one based on the PulseOx study [7], but with some practical differences, particularly in terms of the timing of the screen and response to a positive screen. None of the units required a mandatory echocardiogram as part of the response to a positive screen.

The approach in Australia has been driven in part by some modification of the basic tenants of pulse oximetry screening for CCHD. Whilst the focus in the USA and the UK has been on the implementation of a formal screening program for CCHD, the discussion in Australia and New Zealand has been on the use of the terminology of "Pulse oximetry screening for critical congenital heart disease" versus "Pulse oximetry screening of the well newborn", the timing of pulse oximetry screening, the interpretation and significance of false positives, and the appropriate action for babies who screen positive, all of which have been areas of controversy during the implementation of universal routine pulse oximetry screening in many countries, including the United Kingdom [11].

3. Challenges in Introducing Pulse Oximetry Screening for CCHD

3.1. Screening for CCHD or Documentation of a Vital Sign

Pulse oximetry is used routinely in the assessment of adult patients admitted to hospital. Early warning scores have been developed, inclusive of routine saturation checks, to identify patients before clinical deterioration and preventing admissions to the intensive care unit. Saturation documentation forms part of Paediatric early warning systems, such as the Cardiff and Vale Paediatric Early Warning System and the Melbourne criterion for activation of medical emergency teams [12]. In Australia, local state health authorities have implemented programs such as "Between the Flags" to recognise and respond to patients when their clinical condition starts to deteriorate, which include documenting oxygen saturation [13]. Saturation monitoring has been proposed as an adjunct to the assessment of the newborn in the delivery room and as a routine vital sign assessment [14]. It is proposed that the documentation of oxygen saturation in the newborn should be an integral part of normal vital sign documentation, equivalent in importance to pulse, respirations, heart rate, and blood pressure. Introducing pulse oximetry as part of a routine observational assessment changes the emphasis of a pulse oximetry measure from screening for CCHD (still achieved) to documentation of the fifth vital sign [15]. As a result, it has been our observation that many of the barriers to CCHD screening are minimized, including parental anxiety about the link with CCHD and subsequent refusal of the screen [16], the need to obtain consent in some programs, which can be threatening to parents necessitating an opt-out clause in some countries, including the USA [17], the concept of a false positive for CCHD when the infant has a positive pulse oximetry screen (i.e., is noted to be hypoxic) but is not diagnosed with CCHD, and finally the response to a positive screen, which does not have to be a mandated echocardiogram with all of its resource implications [18].

3.2. Linking 'Pulse Oximetry Screening' to 'Screening for CCHD'

Referring to the screening program as "Pulse oximetry screening of the well newborn" rather than a "Program to screen for critical congenital heart disease" has resulted in better acceptance of the screening program for clinicians and parents in our setting [18]. Pulse oximetry screening identifies some forms of cyanotic heart disease, but does not screen for all CCHD. Some babies with CCHD are missed using pulse oximetry screening, particularly those with obstruction of the aorta. There is a risk of false parental reassurance of absence of congenital heart diseases with the use of the term 'Pulse oximetry screening for CCHD'.

The terminology "Screening for CCHD" may raise anxiety, as it introduces the possibility of a child having a serious health condition. In a recent article by Powell et al. [16] evaluating the acceptability of pulse oximetry screening to mothers, white British and Irish mothers had the lowest rate of decline (5%), while all other minor ethnic groups had an increased likelihood of declining the screening in a research setting (up to 21% in African women). Post-hoc analysis indicated that participants of minor ethnic origin were more anxious, more depressed, less satisfied, and more stressed than the white population who participated in the study. In our opinion, replacing the terminology with "routine pulse oximetry screening" as a documentation of a vital sign undertaken on all babies born in hospital is less likely to raise unnecessary anxiety in parents. The interesting requirement for an opt-out clause in the pulse oximetry screening program in the United States [17] is likely to have resulted from similar observations of parental anxiety.

3.3. Timing of Pulse Oximetry Screening and Significance of False Positives

The AAP work group recommends that screening should not begin until after 24 h of life, or as late as possible if an earlier discharge is planned, and be completed on the second day of life. Dawson et al. [19] have defined reference data for oxygen saturation in healthy full-term infants during their first 24 h of life. The time to reach a stable saturation >95% is generally 20 min in healthy babies (range 3–90 min), so waiting for 24 h is cautious. Earlier screening can lead to more false-positive results because of the transition from fetal to neonatal circulation and the stabilization of systemic oxygen saturation levels [9]. Thangaratinam et al. [8] showed that the false-positive rate for detection of CCHD was particularly low when newborn pulse oximetry was done after 24 h from birth than when it was done before 24 h: 0.05% versus 0.50%. Consequently, many screening programs have chosen to screen after 24 h to decrease the false positives for CCHD. An alternative way of looking at this is that the infants picked up on a positive screening test are infants with low oxygen saturation, regardless of the aetiology, and that any infant with low saturation requires investigation. When the population of infants with a false positive for CCHD are reviewed in the large data sets of screening, more than 50% of them will have important pathology, including congenital pneumonia, sepsis, meconium aspiration syndrome, milder forms of congenital heart disease, and failure to transition (eg. persistent pulmonary hypertension of the newborn (PPHN), transient tachypnea of the newborn (TTN)) [7,20–22]. Although these studies were not specifically designed to assess the cohort of false positives, a false positive result suggests a 'hypoxic' baby and a baby with undiagnosed Group B streptococcal sepsis, pneumonia, or PPHN is just as likely to collapse and die as a baby with undiagnosed CCHD. If documentation of saturation is agreed to be a routine vital sign, are we delaying the documentation of saturation in our babies for the wrong reasons?

When combined with the routine anomaly scan and newborn physical examination, early (4–24 h) pulse oximetry screening adds value to existing screening procedures and is likely to be useful for the identification of cases of CCHD that would otherwise go undetected. The added value in pulse oximetry screening over and above physical examination has been quantitated in two studies. deWahl Granelli [23] showed an increase in sensitivity of CCHD detection from 63% to 83% with specificity remaining at 98%. Similarly, Zhao et al. showed increased sensitivity of CCHD detection from 77.4% to 93.2% with the addition of pulse oximetry screening to the newborn examination [24].

There is clear data to show that infants with CCHD who present collapsed will have a worse neurological outcome than those who are identified before a collapse [3]. As a significant number of infants with CCHD present in the first 24 h with early ductal closure [25], planning a screening program in the first 24 h will result in less collapsed presentations and provide an opportunity for earlier stabilization and intervention. An added benefit is that screening within the first 24 h is less likely to interfere with the discharge process, particularly in those false positive cases that require only minimal intervention, such as a period of observation. The pros and cons of early versus late screening are presented in Table 1.

Table 1. Pros and cons of screening before and after 24 h of age.

<24 h of Age	>24 h of Age
Increased detection of significant and major CHD	Increased detection of significant and major CHD
Optimal for prevention of postnatal hypoxia	Not optimal but still prevents some hypoxic events
Higher false positive rate for CCHD (0.5%)	Lower false positive rate for CCHD (0.05%)
Detection of other pathology (up to 50% of all false positives)	Detection of other pathology (up to 50% of all false positives)
Often still in hospital: doesn't disrupt discharge process	May disrupt discharge process

CHD: congenital heart disease; CCHD: critical congenital heart disease.

3.4. Response to a Positive Screen

The number of false positives for CCHD arising from the physical examination is significantly more than that from pulse oximetry screening [24]. One of the perceived impediments in introducing a pulse oximetry screening program is the need for rapid access to cardiology services to perform an echocardiogram in the event of a failed screening test. In reality, these are babies likely to present to health care providers at some point, apart from the small number with transitional problems that will self-resolve. All health care facilities managing deliveries and newborn babies should already have existing referral and escalation pathways to deal with infants with suspected CHD. Pulse oximetry screening is simply a complement to the existing mechanisms whereby suspected CHD may be identified on physical examination in response to a member of staff reporting a 'dusky' baby or after a low saturation measure during an ad hoc pulse oximetry measure in a dusky appearing baby. These presentations are no different to a 'positive' pulse oximetry screen. In the published pulse oximetry studies, all babies with failed screens were referred for an echocardiogram to allow for full ascertainment of sensitivity and specificity in those babies with a low pulse oximetry reading. In fact, the AAP working group recommended that any newborn with a positive screen result first requires a comprehensive evaluation for causes of hypoxemia. In the absence of other findings to explain hypoxemia, CCHD needs to be excluded on the basis of a diagnostic echocardiogram (which would involve an echocardiogram within the hospital or birthing center or transport to another institution) [9]. The need for an echocardiogram should be determined on a case-by-case basis as it would be for other presentations of potential congenital heart disease (murmur, visible cyanosis). The actual number of infants requiring further investigation as a result of a failed pulse oximetry can be surprisingly small, and in particular the requirement for extra echocardiograms is minimal [18].

4. Pulse Oximetry of the Well Newborn versus Screening for CCHD

The dilemma that many countries are facing when introducing a program to identify hypoxic/borderline hypoxic infants is whether to mandate this as part of a formal national screening program or to introduce pulse oximetry as part of the routine observations performed on a newborn infant. There are pros and cons of each approach and these are summarized in Table 2. The introduction of pulse oximetry for all well newborns prior to discharge, by documenting SpO2 as the 5th vital sign, is appealing and relatively straight forward and the equipment and skills to measure it are already generally available. It is our opinion that delinking the term CCHD from the test allows for the documentation of SpO2 without needing to explain in detail about CCHD and complications that might occur from this, resulting in decreased parental anxiety, a reduced possibility of misinterpretation that CHD has been completely ruled out, false positives becoming less relevant such that earlier screening can be proposed, and a less likely implication of the need for a mandated echocardiogram in the event of a failed screen (Figure 1).

---

1. Consider a pulse oximetry measure as a standard vital sign that needs to be documented in all newborn babies.

2. Delink "Pulse Oximetry Screening" from "Screening for Critical Congenital Heart Diseases" – remove parental anxiety and the perception that CCHD is included / excluded by this test.

3. Measure in the first 24 hrs (allow first 4 hrs for transition). The 'false positives' are actually hypoxic babies warranting evaluation.

4. Do not delay pulse oximetry because an echocardiogram might be required in a false positive (for CCHD) baby.

5. Use existing assessment and referral pathways for a blue baby, heart murmur, and respiratory distress in the local hospital if there is a positive screen. A positive screen needs medical assessment, observation and sometimes a timely echocardiogram as a part of assessment but this is not mandated. We don't have to develop a whole new system.

6. Review the sensitivity and specificity of the current screening processes in place at your institution (antenatal ultrasound and newborn examination), they may be less accurate than introducing pulse oximetry screening

---

Figure 1. Pulse oximetry screening: A new paradigm.

Table 2. Formalised screening program versus vital sign documentation.

Screening Program	Hospital Led/5th Vital Sign
Meeting screening test criteria, Competing with other national screening programs for funding	More easily achievable without a complex application process
Research based: almost 500,000 babies tested	Harder to justify as not linked to CCHD research
Country-wide introduction, mandated, uniformity of coverage	Gaps in provision, Ad Hoc screening
Properly resourced and funded. Quality improvement more easily achieved	Resourcing is not excessive so achievable by most hospitals
CHD is a tested hard outcome	Importance of other diagnoses and timing of the test
Follows existing research based algorithms: reduced flexibility	Delink from CCHD terminology: reduces pressure from false positives and need for echocardiogram.

Importantly, the detailed requirements needed to satisfy inclusion as a formal country-wide screening test are not needed: these requirements can result in significant delays in the introduction of a screening program. The downside of this approach is that there may not be true nationwide screening, particularly at smaller, under-resourced hospitals. The approach may result in a less-uniform approach and lack of a formalized collection of results to understand the impact of screening. In contrast, a formal application to include pulse oximetry screening for CCHD as a part of a country screening program results in proper resourcing, oversight, and governance. It is more likely that all babies at all levels will be screened. However, the process takes time (5 years and still proceeding in the case of the United Kingdom) and will still suffer from all of the issues discussed above when pulse oximetry measures are linked to screening for CCHD. The Nordic countries have been successful in the approach of a hospital-by-hospital introduction of screening, resulting in an overall coverage of screening of close to 100% [26].

5. Conclusions

Currently in our part of the world, Australia has chosen to follow the introduction of screening on a hospital-by-hospital basis, adopting many of the tenants of the 5th vital sign approach, whilst New Zealand has signaled its intention to adopt a country-wide screening program due to some of the unique challenges of health care delivery they have [10]. It will be interesting to track how each country achieves the common aim of improving detection of CCHD and thus reducing deaths and neurodevelopmental injury associated with these significant congenital abnormalities. The body of research to date strongly supports the utility of screening all well newborn infants with pulse oximetry. However, the implementation of screening as performed in the research framework into the real life scenario has been impeded by many of the issues discussed in this paper. As more Units and countries describe their approach to screening and outcomes, a more balanced approach to the introduction of pulse oximetry screening is likely to be achieved.

Conflicts of Interest: The author declares no conflict of interest.

References

1. Hoffman, J.I. It is time for routine neonatal screening by pulse oximetry. *Neonatology* **2011**, *99*, 1–9. [CrossRef] [PubMed]
2. Kuehl, K.S.; Loffredo, C.A.; Ferencz, C. Failure to diagnose congenital heart disease in infancy. *Pediatrics* **1999**, *103*, 743–747. [CrossRef] [PubMed]
3. Snookes, S.H.; Gunn, J.K.; Eldridge, B.J.; Donath, S.M.; Hunt, R.W.; Galea, M.P.; Shekerdemian, L. A systematic review of motor and cognitive outcomes after early surgery for congenital heart disease. *Pediatrics* **2010**, *125*, e818–e827. [CrossRef] [PubMed]
4. Sholler, G.F.; Kasparian, N.A.; Pye, V.E.; Cole, A.D.; Winlaw, D.S. Fetal and post-natal diagnosis of major congenital heart disease: Implications for medical and psychological care in the current era. *J. Paediatr. Child Health* **2011**, *47*, 717–722. [CrossRef] [PubMed]
5. Sharland, G. Fetal cardiac screening: Why bother? *Arch. Dis. Child. Fetal Neonatal Ed.* **2010**, *95*, F64–F68. [PubMed]
6. Mellander, M.; Sunnegardh, J. Failure to diagnose critical heart malformations in newborns before discharge—An increasing problem? *Acta Paediatr.* **2006**, *95*, 407–413. [CrossRef] [PubMed]
7. Ewer, A.K.; Middleton, L.J.; Furmston, A.T.; Bhoyar, A.; Daniels, J.P.; Thangaratinam, S.; Deeks, J.J.; Khan, K.S.; PulseOx Study Group. Pulse oximetry screening for congenital heart defects in newborn infants (pulseox): A test accuracy study. *Lancet* **2011**, *378*, 785–794. [CrossRef]
8. Thangaratinam, S.; Brown, K.; Zamora, J.; Khan, K.S.; Ewer, A.K. Pulse oximetry screening for critical congenital heart defects in asymptomatic newborn babies: A systematic review and meta-analysis. *Lancet* **2012**, *379*, 2459–2464. [CrossRef]
9. Kemper, A.R.; Mahle, W.T.; Martin, G.R.; Cooley, W.C.; Kumar, P.; Morrow, W.R.; Kelm, K.; Pearson, G.D.; Glidewell, J.; Grosse, S.D.; et al. Strategies for implementing screening for critical congenital heart disease. *Pediatrics* **2011**, *128*, e1259–e1267. [CrossRef] [PubMed]
10. Cloete, E.; Gentles, T.L.; Alsweiler, J.M.; Dixon, L.A.; Webster, D.R.; Rowe, D.L.; Bloomfield, F.H. Should new zealand introduce nationwide pulse oximetry screening for the detection of critical congenital heart disease in newborn infants? *N. Z. Med. J.* **2017**, *130*, 64–69. [PubMed]
11. Mikrou, P.; Singh, A.; Ewer, A.K. Pulse oximetry screening for critical congenital heart defects: A repeat UK national survey. *Arch. Dis. Child. Fetal Neonatal Ed.* **2017**, *102*, F558. [CrossRef] [PubMed]
12. Edwards, E.D.; Powell, C.V.; Mason, B.W.; Oliver, A. Prospective cohort study to test the predictability of the cardiff and vale paediatric early warning system. *Arch. Dis. Child.* **2009**, *94*, 602–606. [CrossRef] [PubMed]
13. Health, N. *Children and Infants—Recognition of a Sick Baby or Child in the Emergency Department*; NSW Health: Sydney, Australia, 2011.

14. Katzman, G.H. The newborn's spo2: A routine vital sign whose time has come? *Pediatriks* **1995**, *95*, 161–162. [PubMed]
15. Mower, W.R.; Sachs, C.; Nicklin, E.L.; Baraff, L.J. Pulse oximetry as a fifth pediatric vital sign. *Pediatrics* **1997**, *99*, 681–686. [CrossRef] [PubMed]
16. Powell, R.; Pattison, H.M.; Bhoyar, A.; Furmston, A.T.; Middleton, L.J.; Daniels, J.P.; Ewer, A.K. Pulse oximetry screening for congenital heart defects in newborn infants: An evaluation of acceptability to mothers. *Arch. Dis. Child. Fetal Neonatal Ed.* **2013**, *98*, F59–F63. [CrossRef] [PubMed]
17. Hom, L.A.; Silber, T.J.; Ennis-Durstine, K.; Hilliard, M.A.; Martin, G.R. Legal and ethical considerations in allowing parental exemptions from newborn critical congenital heart disease (cchd) screening. *Am. J. Bioeth.* **2016**, *16*, 11–17. [CrossRef] [PubMed]
18. Bhola, K.; Kluckow, M.; Evans, N. Post-implementation review of pulse oximetry screening of well newborns in an australian tertiary maternity hospital. *J. Paediatr. Child Health* **2014**, *50*, 920–925. [CrossRef] [PubMed]
19. Dawson, J.A.; Vento, M.; Finer, N.N.; Rich, W.; Saugstad, O.D.; Morley, C.J.; Davis, P.G. Managing oxygen therapy during delivery room stabilization of preterm infants. *J. Pediatr.* **2012**, *160*, 158–161. [CrossRef] [PubMed]
20. Narayen, I.C.; Blom, N.A.; Ewer, A.K.; Vento, M.; Manzoni, P.; te Pas, A.B. Aspects of pulse oximetry screening for critical congenital heart defects: When, how and why? *Arch. Dis. Child. Fetal Neonatal Ed.* **2016**, *101*, F162–F167. [CrossRef] [PubMed]
21. Meberg, A.; Brugmann-Pieper, S.; Due, R., Jr.; Eskedal, L.; Fagerli, I.; Farstad, T.; Froisland, D.H.; Sannes, C.H.; Johansen, O.J.; Keljalic, J.; et al. First day of life pulse oximetry screening to detect congenital heart defects. *J. Pediatr.* **2008**, *152*, 761–765. [CrossRef] [PubMed]
22. Arlettaz, R.; Bauschatz, A.S.; Monkhoff, M.; Essers, B.; Bauersfeld, U. The contribution of pulse oximetry to the early detection of congenital heart disease in newborns. *Eur. J. Pediatr.* **2006**, *165*, 94–98. [CrossRef] [PubMed]
23. de-Wahl Granelli, A.; Wennergren, M.; Sandberg, K.; Mellander, M.; Bejlum, C.; Inganas, L.; Eriksson, M.; Segerdahl, N.; Agren, A.; Ekman-Joelsson, B.M.; et al. Impact of pulse oximetry screening on the detection of duct dependent congenital heart disease: A swedish prospective screening study in 39,821 newborns. *Bmj* **2009**, *338*, a3037. [CrossRef] [PubMed]
24. Zhao, Q.M.; Ma, X.J.; Ge, X.L.; Liu, F.; Yan, W.L.; Wu, L.; Ye, M.; Liang, X.C.; Zhang, J.; Gao, Y.; et al. Pulse oximetry with clinical assessment to screen for congenital heart disease in neonates in china: A prospective study. *Lancet* **2014**, *384*, 747–754. [CrossRef]
25. Schultz, A.H.; Localio, A.R.; Clark, B.J.; Ravishankar, C.; Videon, N.; Kimmel, S.E. Epidemiologic features of the presentation of critical congenital heart disease: Implications for screening. *Pediatrics* **2008**, *121*, 751–757. [CrossRef] [PubMed]
26. de-Wahl Granelli, A.; Meberg, A.; Ojala, T.; Steensberg, J.; Oskarsson, G.; Mellander, M. Nordic pulse oximetry screening–implementation status and proposal for uniform guidelines. *Acta Paediatr.* **2014**, *103*, 1136–1142. [CrossRef] [PubMed]

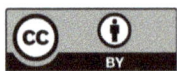

© 2018 by the author. Licensee MDPI, Basel, Switzerland. This article is an open access article distributed under the terms and conditions of the Creative Commons Attribution (CC BY) license (http://creativecommons.org/licenses/by/4.0/).

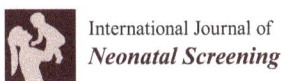

Comment

Comment on Kluckow M. Barriers to the Implementation of Newborn Pulse Oximetry Screening: A Different Perspective.
Int. J. Neonatal Screen. 2018, 4(1), 4

Thomas L. Gentles [1,*], Elza Cloete [2] and Mats Mellander [1,3]

1. Green Lane Paediatric and Congenital Cardiac Service, Starship Children's Hospital, 1023 Auckland, New Zealand; mats.mellander@vgregion.se
2. Liggins Institute, University of Auckland, 1142 Auckland, New Zealand; ElzaC@adhb.govt.nz
3. Queen Silvia Children's Hospital, Department of Pediatric Cardiology, 41650 Gothenburg, Sweden
* Correspondence: tomg@adhb.govt.nz

Received: 29 January 2018; Accepted: 10 April 2018; Published: 14 April 2018

Keywords: pulse oximetry; screening; critical congenital heart disease; neonate

---

We read the review article by Kluckow M (Barriers to the Implementation of Newborn Pulse Oximetry Screening: A Different Perspective. *Int. J. Neonatal Screen.* 2018, 4(1), 4) with interest and agree that this is an important subject to discuss. However, we do not agree with the view as to how pulse oximetry screening for critical congenital heart disease (CCHD) is best implemented and therefore would like to add to this discussion.

The article discusses two important issues in relation to pulse oximetry screening. The first question is whether the oximetry test is better packaged as an assessment of neonatal wellbeing rather than a way to detect CCHD. Kluckow argues for the first alternative as being preferable because he believes this way of doing it causes less anxiety for parents. The second question Kluckow discusses is whether pulse oximetry testing is best delivered as a nationwide screening program or on an individual hospital basis. Kluckow is of the opinion that the second alternative is more likely to be successful (at least in Australia).

If it were not that the first question was closely linked to the second and more important one, the answer would be fairly straightforward, as pulse oximetry testing may detect babies with systemic illness including respiratory illness and infection at a greater rate than it does CCHD [1]. The second question, whether pulse oximetry testing is best delivered as a universal screening program or on an individual basis, is more complex. The answer in part depends on local factors. Who is responsible for the newborn assessment and how would oximetry testing be incorporated into the newborn examination? Who will pay for the time, equipment and disposables? In New Zealand, where the newborn assessment is undertaken by midwives with a number of competing priorities, the incorporation of an oximetry test into the newborn examination is unlikely to be universal. Certainly in a pilot study involving several different hospital care settings, the uptake of oximetry testing ranged between 45% and 85% despite an intensive targeted staff education campaign (preliminary data).

Universal pulse oximetry has the potential to improve health outcomes in the most disadvantaged newborns: those whose mothers are less likely to obtain quality obstetric care and who may not obtain any obstetric care until late in pregnancy [2]. These factors, in addition to maternal obesity, which is also linked to social deprivation, mean that babies of disadvantaged mothers are less likely to have an antenatal diagnosis of CCHD. In New Zealand as elsewhere, a significant number of newborns die or have lasting damage because of the late diagnosis of CCHD [3]. Both New Zealand and Australia have minority indigenous and immigrant populations whose health outcomes fall far below those of the dominant culture. Whichever way the pulse oximetry test is packaged, it is important that its reach and impact are understood and iteratively improved upon. Without an ongoing audit of uptake and knowledge of the population-based (rather than hospital-based) rate of late or undiagnosed CCHD, it is not possible to assess whether a program is effective. An ad hoc roll out of oximetry testing in large tertiary hospitals is likely to target the children of higher income families who are the most likely to have an antenatal diagnosis. Moreover, those born in peripheral hospitals are, in our experience, more likely to receive a delayed diagnosis of CCHD and are therefore most likely to benefit from screening. These same factors are very likely to have contributed to the marked difference in CCHD detection rates in US centers where mandatory screening programs were associated with a 33% reduction in infant death from CCHD compared to no reduction in those states who adopted non-mandatory policies [4]. It is important that these issues are addressed by the broader community to ensure that oximetry testing is delivered in a way that reduces inequity rather than magnifies it.

Neonatal pulse oximetry screening for CCHD has the greatest potential to be effective if implementation is universal. If it is left to each hospital to implement screening, there is a risk that parts of the population who are most likely to benefit from postnatal screening for CCHD will be least likely to receive it.

Conflicts of Interest: The authors declare no conflict of interest.

References

1. Meberg, A. Newborn pulse oximetry screening is not just for heart defects. *Acta Paediatr.* **2015**, *104*, 856–857. [CrossRef] [PubMed]
2. New Zealand Ministry of Health. New Zealand Maternity Clinical Indicators. 2013. Available online: http://www.health.govt.nz/system/files/documents/publications/new-zealand-maternity-clinical-indicators-2013-sep15.pdf (accessed on 25 February 2018).
3. Eckersley, L.; Sadler, L.; Parry, E.; Finucane, K.; Gentles, T.L. Timing of diagnosis affects mortality in critical congenital heart disease. *Arch. Dis. Child.* **2016**, *101*, 516–520. [CrossRef] [PubMed]
4. Abouk, R.; Grosse, S.D.; Ailes, E.C.; Oster, M.E. Association of US State implementation of newborn screening policies for critical congenital heart disease with early infant cardiac death. *JAMA* **2017**, *21*, 2111–2118. [CrossRef] [PubMed]

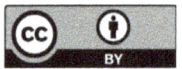

© 2018 by the authors. Licensee MDPI, Basel, Switzerland. This article is an open access article distributed under the terms and conditions of the Creative Commons Attribution (CC BY) license (http://creativecommons.org/licenses/by/4.0/).

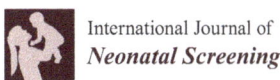 International Journal of
Neonatal Screening

Reply

A Reply to Comment on Kluckow M. Barriers to the Implementation of Newborn Pulse Oximetry Screening: A Different Perspective. *Int. J. Neonatal Screen*. 2018, 4(1), 4

Martin Kluckow

Department of Neonatal Medicine, Royal North Shore Hospital and University of Sydney, Sydney, NSW 2065, Australia; martin.kluckow@sydney.edu.au; Tel.: +61-2-9463-2180

Received: 12 April 2018; Accepted: 13 April 2018; Published: 17 April 2018

The commentary provided by Gentles et al. argues for the implementation of a universal pulse oximetry screening program, and I agree that, if it is possible, this is the optimum way to introduce this important health care measure for all of the reasons set out by the authors. However, there are significant impediments to achieving this in many countries, including in the author's own country of New Zealand, where I understand that several large obstetric hospitals still do not have a full pulse oximetry screening program, pending an attempt at countrywide implementation. One could argue that this is decreasing access to this healthcare intervention, whilst attempting to provide a 100% solution for the whole population. A noble aim, but practically challenging—as has been shown already in the United Kingdom (UK), where, despite one of the world authorities on pulse oximetry screening leading the way towards universal pulse oximetry screening there, it has still not been achieved more than six years after the publication of seminal papers [1]. In fact, most UK hospitals seem to have been adopting the hospital-led screening discussed in my article, with only 19% of hospitals choosing to wait for the National recommendation—if it is achieved [1,2]. I acknowledge that hospital-led screening is a less robust system, but sometimes the gold standard solution is not practical. The issues raised as to time and cost of consumables have been easily overcome in the majority of centres in Australia, at all tiers of health care, as pulse oximetry measurement has become more available and increasingly utilised in postnatal wards for other purposes, apart from formal screening. Audit of the program has been achieved by incorporating screening information into local and national perinatal data collections. The majority of babies born in Australia now undergo pulse oximetry screening. I wish the authors well in achieving their aim of universal pulse oximetry screening in New Zealand.

Conflicts of Interest: The author declares no conflict of interest.

References

1. Mikrou, P.; Singh, A.; Ewer, A.K. Pulse oximetry screening for critical congenital heart defects: A repeat UK national survey. *Arch. Dis. Child. Fetal Neonatal Ed.* **2017**, *102*, F558–F559. [CrossRef] [PubMed]
2. Kluckow, M. Barriers to the Implementation of Newborn Pulse Oximetry Screening: A Different Perspective. *Int. J. Neonatal Screen.* **2018**, *4*, 4. [CrossRef]

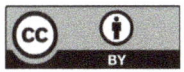 © 2018 by the author. Licensee MDPI, Basel, Switzerland. This article is an open access article distributed under the terms and conditions of the Creative Commons Attribution (CC BY) license (http://creativecommons.org/licenses/by/4.0/).

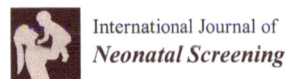 International Journal of
Neonatal Screening

Review

Pulse Oximetry Screening Adapted to a System with Home Births: The Dutch Experience

Ilona C. Narayen [1,*], Nico A. Blom [2] and Arjan B. te Pas [1]

[1] Department of Paediatrics, Division of Neonatology, Leiden University Medical Center, P.O. Box 9200, 2300 RC Leiden, The Netherlands; a.b.te_pas@lumc.nl
[2] Division of Paediatric Cardiology, Leiden University Medical Center, 2333 ZA Leiden, The Netherlands; N.A.Blom@lumc.nl
* Correspondence: i.c.narayen@lumc.nl

Received: 14 January 2018; Accepted: 11 February 2018; Published: 30 March 2018

Abstract: Neonatal screening for critical congenital heart defects is proven to be safe, accurate, and cost-effective. The screening has been implemented in many countries across all continents in the world. However, screening for critical congenital heart defects after home births had not been studied widely yet. The Netherlands is known for its unique perinatal care system with a high rate of home births (18%) and early discharge after an uncomplicated delivery in hospital. We report a feasibility, accuracy, and acceptability study performed in the Dutch perinatal care system. Screening newborns for critical congenital heart defects using pulse oximetry is feasible after home births and early discharge, and acceptable to mothers. The accuracy of the test is comparable to other early-screening settings, with a moderate sensitivity and high specificity.

Keywords: neonates; screening; congenital heart defects; home births

1. Background

To increase the number of timely diagnoses, several studies on screening newborns for critical congenital heart defects (CCHD) using pulse oximetry (PO) have been performed since 2000 and led to an increasing implementation of PO screening across all continents [1,2]. This non-invasive screening method was proven to be reliable, easy to perform, and easy to implement in hospitals. Although studies only investigated the costs, without the long-term benefits, the screening is likely to be cost-effective and studies using questionnaires have shown that the screening was acceptable for parents and caregivers [2–5].

However, all large studies performed so far were in hospital settings and with a postnatal stay of more than five hours. In contrast, The Netherlands has a different perinatal care setting with the highest rate of home births (18%), which are supervised by community midwives [6]. The midwives stay for approximately three hours after birth and come back for their first follow-up visit at day two or three after birth (day of birth is day one). Also, in The Netherlands, mother and newborn are discharged early (within five hours) after uncomplicated vaginal delivery in hospital. For these reasons, the published protocols used in other countries do not match with the Dutch perinatal logistics and it is not possible to extrapolate the results of other PO screening studies to the Dutch perinatal care setting. We therefore performed studies with an adapted PO screening protocol to fit home births and early discharge in the Dutch unique perinatal care setting.

2. Discussion in The Netherlands

After publication of the meta-analysis on PO screening in the Lancet in 2012 it was stated that in The Netherlands it would be difficult to train all 1850 community midwives in performing PO measurements and to provide them all with PO devices [7]. Although the Dutch Association of Pediatricians (NVK) recommends the use of PO in case of resuscitation of a newborn, PO has not been implemented as standard practice in community midwifery [8,9]. The Netherlands has a history of having a high rate of 'natural' deliveries at home, without medical intervention [10]. Community midwives in The Netherlands are traditionally trained in clinical assessment and intervention with little use of technical devices [9]. However, in the Leiden region there is a well-organized clinical and research collaboration between hospitals and community midwives. The midwives participated in a study with recording PO measurements at birth at home. The midwives were trained in one afternoon session and experienced no problems with the use of PO during the study. The study showed that using the PO at home birth was feasible and almost all midwives were enthusiastic about having a PO available, especially in situations with a suboptimal condition of the newborn [9]. We considered the Leiden region the optimal region to pilot PO screening in the Dutch perinatal care setting.

The screening protocol used in the United States and Scandinavia needed to be adapted and made to fit with the visiting scheme of community midwives in The Netherlands [10,11]. Instead of performing one pre- and post-ductal SpO_2 reading 24–48 h after birth, we decided to perform these measurements at two separate time points: the first measurement at least one hour after birth, and the second measurement on day two or three of the newborn's life (day of birth is day one). The first measurement should be performed in the first hours after birth, since community midwives stay for approximately three hours after a delivery and because of discharge within five hours after in-hospital delivery. We were aware that performing screening early (before 24 h) is accompanied with a higher false positive rate due to transitional circulation [2]. However, studies also demonstrated that when the screening was performed after 24 h of life, some CCHD already presented with severe symptoms before the screening was performed [5,12]. The intention of screening is to detect pathology before symptoms occur, making early screening pivotal. Early screening also enables timely detection of other significant pathology, such as infections and respiratory morbidity. We added the second measurement on day two or three of life using the same protocol, at the first follow-up visit of the community midwife, because it is possible that a widely patent ductus arteriosus can cause normal SpO_2 values in newborns with CCHD in the first hours of life. Midwives and nurses were trained in performing and interpreting the PO measurements in a one-day education session. A web-based entry form with an automatic algorithm interpretation was used for quality assurance, and the research team could be reached 24/7 for questions regarding the screening. Handheld pulse oximeters were used for both studies, supplied by Medtronic (Dublin, Ireland). Reusable sensors were used in order to reduce the costs.

3. Pilot Study

We first piloted the adapted protocol in a feasibility study in the Leiden region, in which one academic hospital, two regional hospitals, and 14 midwifery practices are situated [13]. In this study, the Pulse Oximetry Leiden Screening (POLS) study, screening could only be performed after parental consent. Almost all parents who were approached consented and 99% (3059/3090) of the newborns with parental consent were screened. It was reassuring to observe that during the first screening episode in most of the healthy term newborns the pre- and post-ductal SpO_2 was already above 95% in the first hours after birth (10th percentile was 97% pre-ductally and 96% post-ductally within the first hour after birth, $n = 394$). This implies that newborns with SpO_2 values below 95% should be evaluated when they are measured at least one hour after birth. Indeed, in 50% of the newborns with a false positive screening result other morbidities than CCHD were diagnosed, including infections, wet lungs, PPHN, or non-critical congenital heart defects.

4. Acceptability to Mothers

We then assessed the acceptability of performing PO screening at home amongst 1172 mothers participating in the feasibility study by using questionnaire [14]. In this group, screening measurements were performed at least once at home by their community midwife. The response rate was acceptable (77%) and the vast majority (93%) of mothers considered the screening test important for all babies and would recommend the test to someone else.

We concluded that PO screening for CCHD, using the adapted protocol, was feasible in the Dutch perinatal care setting and that screening at home is acceptable to mothers [13,14].

5. Accuracy Study

In order to assess the accuracy of the adapted PO screening, we performed an implementation study in a larger cohort in a much larger region (Leiden–Amsterdam Region (POLAR) study) [15]. This study was carried out in three academic hospitals, 11 regional hospitals and 75 midwifery practices and included 23,959 newborns. The prenatal detection rate was 73% and the sensitivity was 50%, with a specificity of 99%. Four out of five detected CCHD were identified in the first screening test, in the first hours after birth. The fifth CCHD was diagnosed at 12 h after birth, on the day after the date of birth (day 2 of life). Serious illnesses such as infections and respiratory pathology were detected in 61% of all newborns with false positive screening results (Table 1). This study demonstrated that PO screening adapted to home births and early post-delivery hospital discharge contributes to the detection of CCHD in an early, asymptomatic stage. The early detection of CCHD, but also other significant pathologies, such as infections and respiratory morbidity, could be considered as a safety net when newborns are born at home or early discharged after delivery in hospital. In that view, the PO screening has the potential to decrease morbidity and mortality of newborns in The Netherlands.

Table 1. Overview of screening parameters for pilot and accuracy study

	Pilot Study (n = 3059)	Accuracy Study (n = 23,959)
True positive screens, n (%)	0 (0)	5 (0.02)
False negative screens, n (%)	0 (0)	5 (0.02)
False positive screens, n (%)	32 (1.0)	221 (0.9)
Respiratory pathology	8	88
Infection/sepsis	3	31
Non-critical CHD	3	3
Other pathology	2	12
Healthy	16	87

6. Costs

Before screening programs can be recommended for universal implementation, cost effectiveness should be considered. Cost analyses have shown that the PO screening is likely to be cost effective, but only screening in hospitals was taken into account [3,4,16]. The outcome of children after pediatric cardiac surgery has considerably improved in the last decades, but recent data on gained quality-adjusted life years (QALYs) are lacking. However, it is known that a timely diagnosis of CCHD decreases the risk of mortality and morbidity, and also the length of hospital stay [17,18].

In the way our screening was set up, all community midwives would require a pulse oximeter, and positive screenings at home should be transported and referred to hospital. This is likely to increase the costs when performing the screening in the Dutch perinatal care system as compared to settings with deliveries and screening in hospital. Therefore, we also performed a cost-effectiveness analysis with the results of the implementation study. These results will also be published in another article.

7. Prenatal Detection and Sensitivity of PO Screening

PO screening is not a replacement for other screening methods for CCHD, but should be considered as an addition to prenatal screening and physical examination. An early prenatal diagnosis of CCHD allows the parents to be mentally prepared, and gives them the opportunity to terminate the pregnancy. Furthermore, it allows the medical team to prepare a treatment strategy and the delivery can be planned in a congenital heart disease center with a level 3 NICU facility to enable acute surgical or catheter interventions. Prenatal detection varies between countries, and regions within countries, and can be improved with training and logistic interventions [19]. The sensitivity of PO screening is correlated with the prenatal detection rate of CCHD, which ranged from 0 to 82% within performed accuracy studies [20]. Fetal screening, which includes structural anomaly scans, is well organized and highly accessible in The Netherlands; there are strict nationwide requirements regarding the performance of the fetal ultrasounds. Intensive training and audit programs are regionally organized. The prenatal detection rate of CCHD was high in the region where the implementation study was performed [15], but the prenatal detection rate in the other regions of The Netherlands is currently unknown.

Although the overall prenatal detection of CCHD is high, specific defects remain difficult to detect prenatally, such as transposition of the great arteries (TGA), total anomalous pulmonary venous return (TAPVR), pulmonary valve stenosis, aortic valve stenosis, and coarctation of the aorta (CoA) [19,21]. PO screening is efficient at detecting low SpO_2 caused by TGA, TAPVR, and pulmonary valve stenosis, but left-sided obstructive lesions—such as CoA—are frequently missed with PO screening [2,22,23]. It remains challenging to detect CoA in an early stage even in combination with antenatal screening, PO screening and neonatal physical examination. In conclusion, PO is an effective screening method for identifying CCHD, but results of PO screening are correlated with the prenatal detection rate of CCHD. When considering the implementation of PO screening in The Netherlands and anticipating a variable prenatal detection rate in the Dutch regions, the sensitivity is likely to be somewhere between 50% and 70% [15].

8. Comparison with Other Studies

Several studies on PO screening in hospitals were performed which led to implementation in many countries. We performed the first studies, including a feasibility study and a large implementation study, with an adapted protocol for PO screening in a perinatal care system with home births and early postnatal discharge from hospital. Smaller pilot studies on PO screening out-of-hospital settings were performed in the United Kingdom (n = 90) and in the plain community in Wisconsin (n = 440) [24,25]. In The Netherlands, only women with low-risk pregnancies can choose to have a home birth, while in the Plain community in Wisconsin place of birth is not selected based on a risk profile. Instead it is culturally, religiously or financially based and many pregnant women in the Plain community do not receive prenatal screening. The detection of CCHD in this group will probably be higher when compared to our population of home birth deliveries.

This was the first screening set up where two separate screening episodes were used. Also, the first screening moment was earlier when compared to other early screening studies (8, 30). In general, it is not recommended to perform PO screening in the first hours after birth, because of the probability of having a higher false positive rate due to transitional circulation. In our Leiden pilot study, however, we demonstrated that SpO_2 values in healthy newborns were above 95% within the first hour of life [13].

9. Current Status

After finalizing the studies, a large number of caregivers did not want to await a governmental decision regarding top-down universal implementation, which can take several years. Bottom-up implementation has already begun in the studied region using the logistics that was set up for the study; the screening is continued in all participating hospitals in the POLAR study, as well as by 36% of all participating community midwifery practices, and this rate is still increasing. The perinatal caregivers in these hospitals and practices were convinced of the usefulness of PO screening.

10. Conclusions

PO screening for CCHD is feasible to perform and acceptable to mothers in the Dutch perinatal care setting with an adapted protocol for home births and early postnatal discharge from hospital. The screening detects CCHD at an early symptomatic stage with the extra benefit of detecting other significant and potentially life-threatening morbidities, such as infections and respiratory pathology. Implementation of PO screening for CCHD and other morbidities has the potential to decrease infant morbidity and mortality and increase the safety of newborns born at home or discharged from hospital in the first hours of life.

Author Contributions: Ilona C. Narayen performed literature review and analysis, wrote the first draft of the article, and gave final approval for publication of the report. Nico A. Blom supervised the writing of the report, reviewed and edited the manuscript, and gave final approval for publication of the report. Arjan B. te Pas supervised the analysis and writing of the article, reviewed and edited the manuscript, and gave final approval for publication of the report.

Conflicts of Interest: The authors declare no conflict of interest.

References

1. Hom, L.A.; Martin, G.R. U.S. international efforts on critical congenital heart disease screening: Can we have a uniform recommendation for Europe? *Early Hum. Dev.* **2014**, *90*, S11–S14. [CrossRef]
2. Thangaratinam, S.; Brown, K.; Zamora, J.; Khan, K.S.; Ewer, A.K. Pulse oximetry screening for critical congenital heart defects in asymptomatic newborn babies: A systematic review and meta-analysis. *Lancet* **2012**, *379*, 2459–2464. [CrossRef]
3. Peterson, C.; Grosse, S.D.; Oster, M.E.; Olney, R.S.; Cassell, C.H. Cost-effectiveness of routine screening for critical congenital heart disease in US newborns. *Pediatrics* **2013**, *132*, e595–e603. [CrossRef] [PubMed]
4. Roberts, T.E.; Barton, P.M.; Auguste, P.E.; Middleton, L.J.; Furmston, A.T.; Ewer, A.K. Pulse oximetry as a screening test for congenital heart defects in newborn infants: A cost-effectiveness analysis. *Arch. Dis. Child.* **2012**, *97*, 221–226. [CrossRef] [PubMed]
5. Ewer, A.K.; Furmston, A.T.; Middleton, L.J.; Deeks, J.J.; Daniels, J.P.; Pattison, H.M.; Powell, R.; Roberts, T.E.; Barton, P.; Auguste, P.; et al. Pulse oximetry as a screening test for congenital heart defects in newborn infants: A test accuracy study with evaluation of acceptability and cost-effectiveness. *Health Technol. Assess.* **2012**, *16*, 1–184. [CrossRef] [PubMed]
6. Netherlands Statistics; CBS Statline. Delivery and Birth: 1989–2015; Netherlands Statistics: The Hague, The Netherlands. Available online: http://statline.cbs.nl/Statweb/publication/?DM=SLNL&PA=81628NED&D1=0-22&D2=a&VW=T (accessed on 7 April 2017).
7. De Visser, E. Hartonderzoek BIJ Baby's Effectief. *Volkskrant*, 2 May 2012.
8. Nederlandse Vereniging voor Kindergeneesunde. Richtlijn Reanimatie van Het Kind BIJ de Geboorte. 2014. Available online: http://www.nvk.nl/Portals/0/richtlijnen/reanimatie/Reanimatie%20van%20het%20kind%20bij%20de%20geboorte_%20NVK%20richtlijn%202014_revisie%2011%20dec%202014.pdf (accessed on 7 April 2017).
9. Smit, M.; Ganzeboom, A.; Dawson, J.A.; Walther, F.J.; Bustraan, J.; van Roosmalen, J.J.; te Pas, A.B. Feasibility of pulse oximetry for assessment of infants born in community based midwifery care. *Midwifery* **2014**, *30*, 539–543. [CrossRef] [PubMed]
10. Kemper, A.R.; Mahle, W.T.; Martin, G.R.; Cooley, W.C.; Kumar, P.; Morrow, W.R.; Kelm, K.; Pearson, G.D.; Glidewell, J.; Grosse, S.D.; et al. Strategies for implementing screening for critical congenital heart disease. *Pediatrics* **2011**, *128*, e1259–e1267. [CrossRef] [PubMed]
11. Narayen, I.C.; Blom, N.A.; Verhart, M.S.; Smit, M.; Posthumus, F.; van den Broek, A.J.; Havers, H.; Haak, M.C.; te Pas, A.B. Adapted protocol for pulse oximetry screening for congenital heart defects in a country with homebirths. *Eur. J. Pediatr.* **2015**, *174*, 129–132. [CrossRef] [PubMed]
12. De-Wahl Granelli, A.; Wennergren, M.; Sandberg, K.; Mellander, M.; Bejlum, C.; Inganas, L.; Eriksson, M.; Segerdahl, N.; Agren, A.; Ekman-Joelsson, B.M.; et al. Impact of pulse oximetry screening on the detection of duct dependent congenital heart disease: A Swedish prospective screening study in 39,821 newborns. *BMJ* **2009**, *338*, a3037. [CrossRef] [PubMed]

13. Narayen, I.C.; Blom, N.A.; Bourgonje, M.S.; Haak, M.C.; Smit, M.; Posthumus, F.; van den Broek, A.J.; Havers, H.M.; te Pas, A.B. Pulse Oximetry Screening for Critical Congenital Heart Disease after Home Birth and Early Discharge. *J. Pediatr.* **2016**, *170*, 188–192. [CrossRef] [PubMed]
14. Narayen, I.C.; Kaptein, A.A.; Hogewoning, J.A.; Blom, N.A.; te Pas, A.B. Maternal acceptability of pulse oximetry screening at home after home birth or very early discharge. *Eur. J. Pediatr.* **2017**, *176*, 669–672. [CrossRef] [PubMed]
15. Narayen, I.C.; Blom, N.A.; van Geloven, N.; Blankman, E.I.; van den Broek, A.J.M.; Bruijn, M.; Clur, S.B.; van den Dungen, F.A.; Havers, H.M.; van Laerhoven, H.; et al. Accuracy of pulse oximetry screening for critical congenital heart defects after home birth and early postnatal discharge. *J. Pediatr.* **2018**. [CrossRef] [PubMed]
16. Griebsch, I.; Knowles, R.L.; Brown, J.; Bull, C.; Wren, C.; Dezateux, C.A. Comparing the clinical and economic effects of clinical examination, pulse oximetry, and echocardiography in newborn screening for congenital heart defects: A probabilistic cost-effectiveness model and value of information analysis. *Int. J. Technol. Assess. Health Care* **2007**, *23*, 192–204. [CrossRef] [PubMed]
17. Brown, K.L.; Ridout, D.A.; Hoskote, A.; Verhulst, L.; Ricci, M.; Bull, C. Delayed diagnosis of congenital heart disease worsens preoperative condition and outcome of surgery in neonates. *Heart* **2006**, *92*, 1298–1302. [CrossRef] [PubMed]
18. Peterson, C.; Dawson, A.; Grosse, S.D.; Riehle-Colarusso, T.; Olney, R.S.; Tanner, J.P.; Kirby, R.S.; Correia, J.A.; Watkins, S.M.; Cassell, C.H. Hospitalizations, costs, and mortality among infants with critical congenital heart disease: How important is timely detection? *Birth Defects Res. A Clin. Mol. Teratol.* **2013**, *97*, 664–672. [CrossRef] [PubMed]
19. Van Velzen, C.L.; Clur, S.A.; Rijlaarsdam, M.E.; Bax, C.J.; Pajkrt, E.; Heymans, M.W.; Bekker, M.N.; Hruda, J.; de Groot, C.J.; Blom, N.A.; et al. Prenatal detection of congenital heart disease—Results of a national screening programme. *BJOG* **2016**, *123*, 400–407. [CrossRef] [PubMed]
20. Narayen, I.C.; Blom, N.A.; Ewer, A.K.; Vento, M.; Manzoni, P.; te Pas, A.B. Aspects of pulse oximetry screening for critical congenital heart defects: When, how and why? *Arch. Dis. Child. Fetal Neonatal Ed.* **2016**, *101*, F162–F167. [CrossRef] [PubMed]
21. Van Velzen, C.L.; Clur, S.A.; Rijlaarsdam, M.E.; Pajkrt, E.; Bax, C.J.; Hruda, J.; de Groot, C.J.; Blom, N.A.; Haak, M.C. Prenatal diagnosis of congenital heart defects: Accuracy and discrepancies in a multicenter cohort. *Ultrasound Obstet Gynecol.* **2016**, *47*, 616–622. [CrossRef] [PubMed]
22. Ewer, A.K. Evidence for CCHD screening and its practical application using pulse oximetry. *Early Hum. Dev.* **2014**, *90*, S19–S21. [CrossRef]
23. Riede, F.T.; Schneider, P. Most wanted, least found: Coarctation. *Neonatology* **2012**, *101*, 13. [CrossRef] [PubMed]
24. Cawsey, M.J.; Noble, S.; Cross-Sudworth, F.; Ewer, A.K. Feasibility of pulse oximetry screening for critical congenital heart defects in homebirths. *Arch. Dis. Child. Fetal Neonatal Ed.* **2016**, *101*, F349–F351. [CrossRef] [PubMed]
25. Lhost, J.J.; Goetz, E.M.; Belling, J.D.; van Roojen, W.M.; Spicer, G.; Hokanson, J.S. Pulse oximetry screening for critical congenital heart disease in planned out-of-hospital births. *J. Pediatr.* **2014**, *165*, 485–489. [CrossRef] [PubMed]

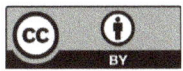

© 2018 by the authors. Licensee MDPI, Basel, Switzerland. This article is an open access article distributed under the terms and conditions of the Creative Commons Attribution (CC BY) license (http://creativecommons.org/licenses/by/4.0/).

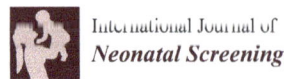

Review

Pulse Oximetry Screening in Germany—Historical Aspects and Future Perspectives

Frank-Thomas Riede [1,*], Christian Paech [1] and Thorsten Orlikowsky [2]

1 Department of Paediatric Cardiology, Heart Centre, University of Leipzig, 04289 Leipzig, Strümpellstr. 39, Germany; christian.paech@medizin.uni-leipzig.de
2 Department of Neonatology, University Childrens Hospital Aachen, 52072 Aachen, Pauwelsstr. 30, Germany; torlikowsky@ukaachen.de
* Correspondence: frank-thomas.riede@medizin.uni-leipzig.de

Received: 31 March 2018; Accepted: 23 April 2018; Published: 28 April 2018

Abstract: In January 2017, pulse oximetry screening was legally implemented in routine neonatal care in Germany. The preceding developments, which were the prerequisite for this step, are described in the specific context of Germany's health care system. Continued evaluation of the method is imperative and may lead to modifications in the screening protocol, ideally in accordance with the efforts in other countries.

Keywords: critical congenital heart disease; pulse oximetry screening; Germany

1. Historical Aspects: From Clinical Data

The most severe, life-threatening forms of congenital heart disease (CHD) requiring intervention very early in life are termed critical (CCHD). During the last decades of the past century, advances in surgical techniques, as well as in perioperative intensive care medicine, led to an improved survival of neonates with CCHD but further progress is likely to be limited.

Delayed diagnosis of CCHD with its potential of cardiac collapse and even death has long been recognized, but its relative importance increased only with the above-mentioned developments. In Germany, Prof. P. Schneider, the former head of the department of Paediatric Cardiology at the Leipzig Heart Centre, described addressing the postnatal diagnostic gap in CCHD as a challenge not only for paediatric cardiologists but for all involved in perinatal care, thus requiring an interdisciplinary and collaborative approach [1].

The first step was to increase the awareness of the problem by establishing and participating in regional educational programs for paediatricians, neonatologists and midwives, starting in the first years of the last decade. Although data from the literature at that time was very limited, using pulse oximetry screening to reduce the diagnostic gap in CCHD has been informally proposed in light of its well-known advantages (availability, ease of use, non-invasiveness, and low cost) [1–4].

A survey in Saxony (the federal state in which the Leipzig Heart Centre is situated) revealed that in January 2006, 62% (n = 29) of all responding perinatal and neonatal units (n = 47; response rate 92%) used pulse oximetry screening regularly. Thus, the prerequisites were ideal to perform a prospective multicentre study on pulse oximetry screening. In the study population, the prenatal detection rate of CCHD was comparatively high (60%). However, there was still a diagnostic gap of 20%, which could be reduced to 4.4% by pulse oximetry screening [5]. Based on the data from this study, the working Groups for Perinatology and Neonatology of the Saxonian Medical Association recommended the implementation of pulse oximetry screening in routine care in October 2009. At around the same time, Tautz et al. published their experience with pulse oximetry screening paralleled by the large series from Norway and Sweden [6–8].

In December 2009, a nationwide survey on pulse oximetry screening in Germany was conducted. A questionnaire was sent to all 890 perinatal and neonatal units; the response rate was 29% ($n = 255$). In 46% of the responding units, pulse oximetry screening had already been established. Although, in the majority of cases, it had only been established in the last three years. However, the percentage of units performing pulse oximetry screening showed remarkable regional differences, possibly at least in part related to the regional effects of the activities in Saxony (Figure 1).

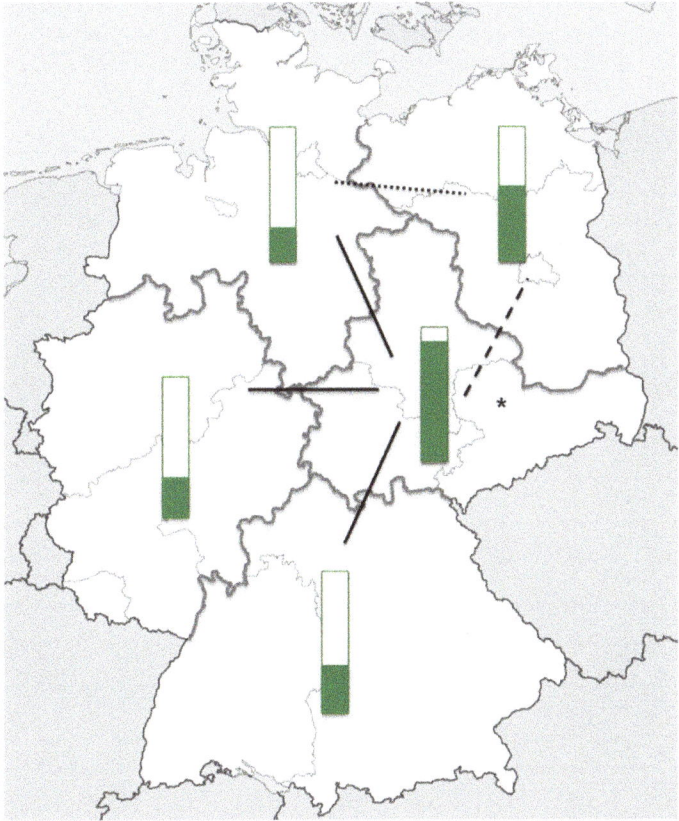

Figure 1. Pulse oximetry screening in Germany in December 2009. Green bars indicate the percentage of perinatal and neonatal units performing pulse oximetry screening as per December 2009 in five regions in Germany. The black lines indicate the level of significance (dotted line: $p < 0.05$, dashed line: $p < 0.01$, solid line, $p < 0.001$). The asterisk indicates the federal state of Saxony. Source of the map: adaptation from svg/2000px-Germany_location_map.svg.png; author: NordNordWest; http://creativecommons.org/licenses/by-sa/3.0/de/legalcode.

Another interesting finding was to reveal of differences in the use of pulse oximetry screening depending on the level of perinatal care. The latter had been defined in Germany in 2006 in an attempt to centralize the management of risk pregnancies and extreme prematurity (Table 1). Pulse oximetry screening was used less in obstetrical clinics (Figure 2). This may, in part, be explained by the expected low risk profile for pregnancies and neonates in these units. Yet, as existing strategies failed to completely predict CCHD, pulse oximetry screening may be especially useful in these settings.

Table 1. Levels of neonatal care in Germany (modified after [9,10]).

Level of Care	Admission Criteria
Perinatal centre level 1	Expected prematurity with a birth weight of <1250 g or a gestational age of <29 weeks triplet pregnancy and gestational age <33 weeks; multiple pregnancy Prenatal diagnosis of any fetal or maternal condition necessitating immediate postnatal intensive care (critical congenital heart disease, diaphragmatic hernia, myelomeningocele, gastroschisis)
Perinatal centre level 2	Expected prematurity with a birth weight of 1250–1499 g or a gestational age of $\geq$29 to <32 weeks HELLP syndrome Intrauterine growth restriction <3rd percentile Insulin-dependent gestational diabetes with elevated risk for the fetus/newborn
Perinatal clinic	Expected prematurity with a birth weight of $\geq$1500 g or a gestational age of $\geq$32 to <36 weeks Intrauterine growth restriction between third and tenth percentile Insulin-dependent gestational diabetes without elevated risk for the fetus/newborn
Obstetrical clinic	Gestational age $\geq$36 weeks, uncomplicated delivery expected

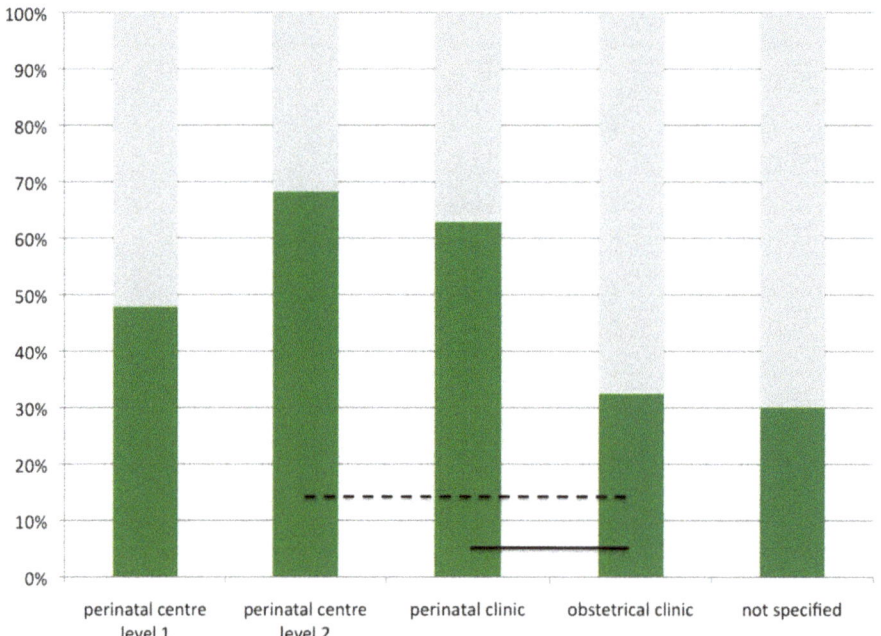

Figure 2. Pulse oximetry screening and level of neonatal care. Green bars indicate percentage of units using pulse oximetry screening as per December 2009 in Germany. Black lines indicate level of significance (dashed line: $p < 0.01$, solid line, $p < 0.001$).

In light of the increasing body of evidence on the benefits of pulse oximetry screening [11,12], the German Society for Paediatric Cardiology supported the use of pulse oximetry screening in 2011 and formulated a statement with recommendations for practical aspects of its implementation in 2013 [13,14]. Likewise, the German Society for Neonatology and Paediatric intensive care (GNPI) recommended the use of pulse oximetry screening in its guidelines for neonatal care in 2012 [15]. However, the effects of these nonbinding recommendations remained unknown.

2. To Legal Regulation

In the nationwide survey of 2009 only 26% of perinatal and neonatal units considered it necessary to have legal regulations in place, in case pulse oximetry screening should be implemented. However, patient representatives had a different view. A group led by the "Bundesverband herzkranke Kinder" (BVHK) initiated the development of a legal regulation.

Germany's national health care insurance system, introduced in 1883, has been highly regulated. Since 1975, more than 90% of the population have been enrolled in the statutory health insurance, the remaining 10% have been nearly completely covered by private or other health insurance [16]. Thus, regulations concerning the scope of health care services provided by insurers affect almost the entire population.

The regulation of medical care and the implementation of legal requirements on new drugs and methods of treatment by directives are the central tasks of a federal committee (Gemeinsamer Bundesausschuss, G-BA). It was established in January 2004 as the highest decision-making body of the joint self-administration of physicians, dentists, psychotherapists, hospitals and health insurance providers.

Preventive examinations and screening tests in neonates are regulated in the Directive on Early Detection of Diseases in Children up to the age of six years. Currently, each newborn is entitled to three examinations immediately after birth (U1), between the third and tenth day of life (U2), and at the end of (or early after) the neonatal period (fourth to fifth week of life, U3). Extended metabolic screening, hearing screening (since 2009), an ultrasound of the hips and the Brückner test (fundoscopy, since 2016) are also included.

The implementation of a new method requires a formal consultation process and a subsequent positive resolution by the G-BA. The initiation of such a process may be requested by independent members of the G-BA, by health insurers, the Association of Statutory Health Insurance Physicians, the corresponding association of dentists, the German Hospital Society and patient representatives, but not by physicians or medical professional societies.

In September 2012, the group of patient representatives mentioned above submitted an application at the G-BA to initiate a consultation process on pulse oximetry screening, which was granted in November 2012. In June 2013, an independent scientific organisation, the Institute for Quality and Cost Effectiveness in Health Care (Institut für Qualität und Wirtschaftlichkeit im Gesundheitswesen, IQWiG), was commissioned with a detailed analysis of the possible effects of pulse oximetry screening in the current setting of peri- and neonatal care in Germany. The evaluation was mainly based on available data from the literature, but statements from experts, national medical professional associations, and patient representatives were also included. In its final report, published in May 2015, the IQWiG concluded that current evidence suggests a benefit of pulse oximetry screening as an adjunct to the pre-existing diagnostic standard (U1 and U2) with respect to the timely diagnosis of CCHD in neonates [17].

In January 2017, after an internal evaluation of the IQWiG's report, statements from experts and medical professional associations, a decree of the G-BA was published, announcing the implementation of pulse oximetry screening in routine neonatal care in Germany [18].

The algorithm for pulse oximetry screening, as recommended by the G-BA, is shown in Figure 3. In most aspects, it is similar to the one used in the German multicentre study, published by one of the authors in 2010 [5]. However, an important difference lies in the role of echocardiography. According to the current recommendations, echocardiography may be omitted if another cause of hypoxia is found. This approach may be reasonable especially when a positive pulse oximetry screening draws attention to clinical signs suggesting other neonatal pathologies such as pneumonia or sepsis, cases in which echocardiography would only delay appropriate diagnosis and treatment.

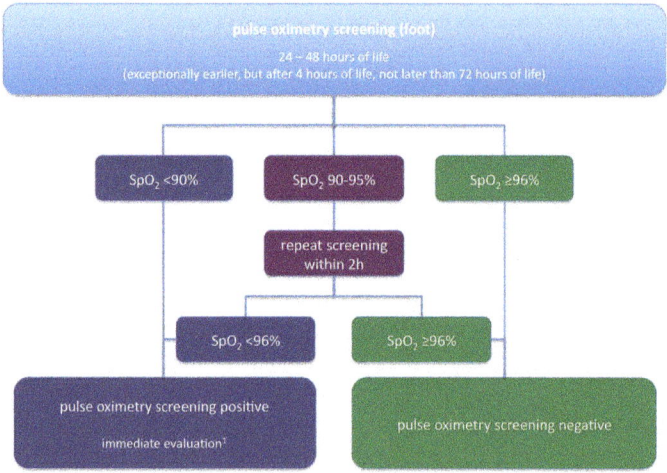

Figure 3. Algorithm for pulse oximetry screening in Germany as recommended by the Common Federal Committee (Gemeinsamer Bundesausschuss, G-BA), modified after [19] by a specialist in paediatrics, ideally with subspecialty training in neonatology/paediatric cardiology.

3. Future Perspectives

As per the decree of the G-BA, the quality and efficacy of pulse oximetry screening in Germany are going to be evaluated after its implementation. By no later than 31 December 2018, an independent scientific institution will be assigned to perform an analysis on the basis of a representative sample to answer a defined set of target parameters (Table 2). However, further aspects might also prove relevant and be included (Table 3).

Table 2. Target parameters for the evaluation of pulse oximetry screening after its implementation in Germany as defined by the G-BA [18].

Number and Percentage of Newborns
- having received pulse oximetry screening
- with a negative screening result on the first measurement ($SpO_2 \geq 96\%$)
- with a positive screening result on the first measurement ($SpO_2 < 90\%$)
- with an abnormal result on the first measurement with the need to repeat the test (SpO_2 90–95%)
- with a negative screening result on the second measurement ($SpO_2 \geq 96\%$)
- with a positive screening result on the second measurement ($SpO_2 < 96\%$)
- referred to a paediatrician/neonatologist
False positive results
Number of newborns with CCHD detected by pulse oximetry screening
Timing of diagnostic and therapeutic procedures in newborns with CCHD

Table 3. Possible additional target parameters for the evaluation of pulse oximetry screening after its implementation in Germany.

Number and Percentage of Newborns
- with a prenatal diagnosis of CCHD
- with diagnosis of CCHD based on clinical signs/physical examination before pulse oximetry screening
False negative results
Detection of neonatal diseases in newborns with false positive screening results (with respect to CCHD)
Reasons for not performing pulse oximetry screening in eligible newborns

Screening is definitely better than no screening, and despite the fact that the national screening program will hopefully increase the early detection of CCHD systematically, several controversies will remain with respect to the time of screening, cut off-values, and the follow-up algorithm.

In comparison to the algorithm in the UK, suggesting an early screening before 24 h of age [11], the German, as well as the American algorithm, recommend screening between 24 h and 48 h of age as the "best screening window" [19,20]. The G-BA states that screening may be performed "in exceptional cases at the earliest of four hours after birth" to account for infants discharged from hospital within 24 h after birth. In most published data on screening before 24 h of age, the rate of false positives was up to 10 times higher (0.8% vs. 0.05%) [21]. In this respect, "false positive" means, "false test positive", i.e., no CCHD detectable in the follow-up. Nevertheless, early screening before 24 h identified more non-cardiac diseases (sepsis, persistent pulmonary hypertension of the newborn) at an early stage before newborns were symptomatic. In the German study, 18 of the 36 newborns with CCHD (50%) showed symptoms before screening [5], which is the very situation that screening aims to prevent. Thus, earlier screening might be desirable from both the neonatologist's and the paediatric cardiologist's perspective. However, the impact of pulse oximetry screening on the detection of noncardiac disease has not been evaluated systematically yet. Expanding the spectrum of target parameters for analysis of efficacy of pulse oximetry screening, as determined by the G-BA (Table 2) by additional parameters (Table 3), might provide appropriate data and allow for evidence-based modifications of the screening algorithm so that early screening and a timely diagnosis can be counterbalanced with the false positive rate. Nevertheless, one has to bear in mind that the problem of severe cardiovascular compromise related to CCHD cannot be completely avoided, neither by thorough clinical examination, nor by pulse oximetry, and not even by prenatal diagnosis. This is because for example, in neonates with hypoplastic left heart syndrome or transposition of the great arteries with restrictive or closed foramen ovale, symptoms may occur despite immediate and appropriate treatment.

Modification of the upper time limit for screening might also become necessary. The German algorithm specifies, that the screening may be performed no later than after the 2nd check-up by the paediatrician. Newborns who have already been discharged at that age, receive their standard investigation (U2) from a paediatrician either in his office or at home. This check-up has to be performed between the third and the tenth day of life. In these cases, if early screening has not been performed, substantial risk for falling into a diagnostic gap remains. Furthermore, it would be necessary for all paediatricians to use portable saturation devices for their outpatient visits (U2). For newborns born at home, midwives would have to be trained systematically.

It would be desirable that pulse oximetry screening for the detection of CCHD is recommended for all European countries. A consensus statement on its implementation includes that it should be performed with new-generation equipment that is motion tolerant, after 6 h of life or before discharge from the birthing centre (preferably within 24 h after birth), and should be done in two extremities, the right hand and either foot [22].

The majority of studies used saturations from one post ductal site—either foot. Recently, studies have employed saturations from two sites—the right hand and one foot—giving both pre- and post-ductal saturations. Therefore, rather than a single absolute saturation leading to the test result, two individual values, and also the difference between the two, contribute to the result. Although a systematic review did not identify a significant difference in sensitivity between the two methods [21], this may be explained by the preponderance of single measurement, and further analyses are necessary.

Post hoc analysis of the raw data revealed that post ductal only measurement would miss a small but significant proportion of babies that dual testing would identify [23]. This may become important in Germany considering the birth rate of approximately 800,000 per year.

In contrast to many other studies from the UK and the USA, the cut-off value was chosen to be 96%, following the experiences of the German trial [5]. Other rather big one-step screening studies used 95%. Whether this single point of saturation difference really makes a difference in specificity or false positives remains to be evaluated. However, combining regional or national studies in Europe in meta-analyses, maybe resulting in a common algorithm, is hampered by different thresholds and procedures. For example, all authors recommending a two-site screening use different combinations of thresholds and differences between measurement sites for definition of a positive screening result [7,9,20].

Prenatal echocardiography has the potential to detect virtually all forms of CCHD up to the point where, in single institutions, pulse oximetry screening for CCHD becomes ineffective [24]. Being highly dependent on operator experience and appropriate technical equipment, which are neither widely available, nor will be in the near future, prenatal detection rates in larger regions or countries remain substantially lower [25]. In Germany, the rate of prenatal diagnoses for all CHD has been 12%, ranging from approximately 5 to 68% in CCHD, depending on the type of lesion [26]. In 2013, completion of a four-chamber view has been implemented in routine pregnancy care by the G-BA. It has been estimated that this may ameliorate the prenatal detection rate up to 30–40%, concluding that pulse oximetry screening will be able to substantially contribute to a timely diagnosis of CCDH in the years to come [17].

A recent U.S. study has shown a substantial reduction of mortality from undiagnosed CCHD after the implementation of pulse oximetry screening [27]. In populations where mortality from undiagnosed CCHD was low before the introduction of pulse oximetry screening, a comparable effect might be expected on the reduction of severe morbidity in affected neonates [5,28].

4. Conclusions

In the past decade, pulse oximetry screening in Germany has made its way from clinical trials to the statutory introduction into clinical routine as an adjunct to prenatal diagnosis and clinical examination. This will hopefully further improve the prognosis of infants with CCHD. Continuing evaluation of its effectiveness is necessary to allow for modifications of the screening protocol when appropriate.

Author Contributions: F.-T.R. and T.O. conceived and designed the work. C.P. thoroughly revised the manuscript.

Acknowledgments: We thank Andy Ewer for his advice on creating the manuscript. We are grateful to Franziska Wagner for language editing of the manuscript. There is no funding to be disclosed.

Conflicts of Interest: The authors declare no conflict of interest.

References

1. Schneider, P.; Kostelka, M.; Kändler, L.; Möckel, A.; Riede, F.T.; Dähnert, I. Die diagnostische Lücke bei neonatalen Herzerkrankungen—Herausforderung für Neonatologie und Kinderkardiologie. *Kinder und Jugendmed.* **2004**, *4*, 188–193. [CrossRef]
2. Bakr, A.F.; Habib, H.S. Combining Pulse Oximetry and Clinical Examination in Screening for Congenital Heart Disease. *Pediatr. Cardiol.* **2005**, *26*, 832–835. [CrossRef] [PubMed]
3. Hoke, T.R.; Donohue, P.K.; Bawa, P.K.; Mitchell, R.D.; Pathak, A.; Rowe, P.C.; Byrne, B.J. Oxygen Saturation as a Screening Test for Critical Congenital Heart Disease: A Preliminary Study. *Pediatr. Cardiol.* **2002**, *23*, 403–409. [CrossRef] [PubMed]
4. Koppel, R.I.; Druschel, C.M.; Carter, T.; Goldberg, B.E.; Mehta, P.N.; Talwar, R.; Bierman, F.Z. Effectiveness of Pulse Oximetry Screening for Congenital Heart Disease in Asymptomatic Newborns. *Pediatrics* **2003**, *111*, 451–455. [CrossRef] [PubMed]
5. Riede, F.T.; Wörner, C.; Dähnert, I.; Möckel, A.; Kostelka, M.; Schneider, P. Effectiveness of neonatal pulse oximetry screening for detection of critical congenital heart disease in daily clinical routine—Results from a prospective multicenter study. *Eur J. Pediatr.* **2010**, *169*, 975–981. [CrossRef] [PubMed]
6. Meberg, A.; Brügmann-Pieper, S.; Due, R., Jr.; Eskedal, L.; Fagerli, I.; Farstad, T.; Frøisland, D.H.; Sannes, C.H.; Johansen, O.J.; Keljalic, J.; et al. First Day of Life Pulse Oximetry Screening to Detect Congenital Heart Defects. *J. Pediatr.* **2008**, *152*, 761–765. [CrossRef] [PubMed]

7. De-Wahl Granelli, A.; Wennergren, M.; Sandberg, K.; Mellander, M.; Bejlum, C.; Inganäs, L.; Eriksson, M.; Segerdahl, N.; Agren, A.; Ekman-Joelsson, B.M.; et al. Impact of pulse oximetry screening on the detection of duct dependent congenital heart disease: A Swedish prospective screening study in 39,821 newborns. *BMJ* **2009**, *338*, a3037. [CrossRef] [PubMed]
8. Tautz, J.; Merkel, C.; Loersch, F.; Egen, O.; Hägele, F.; Thon, H.M.; Schaible, T. Implication of pulse oxymetry screening for detection of congenital heart defects. *Klin. Padiatr.* **2010**, *222*, 291–295. [CrossRef] [PubMed]
9. Bekanntmachung eines Beschlusses des Gemeinsamen Bundesausschusses nach §91 Abs. 7 des Fünften Buches Sozialgesetzbuch (SGB V) zur Vereinbarung über Maßnahmen zur Qualitätssicherung der Versorgung von Früh- und Neugeborenen nach §137 Abs. 1 Satz 3 Nr. 2 SGB V. Gemeinsamer Bundesausschuss. Available online: https://www.g-ba.de/downloads/39-261-229/2005-09-20-Vereinbarung-Frueh_Neu.pdf (accessed on 31 March 2018).
10. Richtlinie des Gemeinsamen Bundesausschusses über Maßnahmen zur Qualitätssicherung der Versorgung von Früh- und Reifgeborenen. Gemeinsamer Bundesausschuss. Available online: https://www.g-ba.de/downloads/62-492-1487/QFR-RL_2017-10-19_iK-2018-01-01.pdf (accessed on 20 March 2018).
11. Ewer, A.K.; Middleton, L.J.; Furmston, A.T.; Bhoyar, A.; Daniels, J.P.; Thangaratinam, S.; Deeks, J.J.; Khan, K.S. Pulse oximetry screening for congenital heart defects in newborn infants (PulseOx): A test accuracy study. *Lancet* **2011**, *378*, 785–794. [CrossRef]
12. Turska Kmieć, A.; Borszewska Kornacka, M.K.; Błaż, W.; Kawalec, W.; Zuk, M. Early screening for critical congenital heart defects in asymptomatic newborns in Mazovia province: Experience of the POLKARD pulse oximetry programme 2006–2008 in Poland. *Kardiol. Pol.* **2012**, *70*, 370–376. [PubMed]
13. Abdul-Khaliq, H.; Berger, F. Die Diagnose wird häufig zu spät gestellt. *Dtsch. Arztebl.* **2011**, *108*, A1684.
14. Lindinger, A.; Dähnert, I.; Riede, F.T. Stellungnahme zum Pulsoximetrie-Screening zur Erfassung von Kritischen Angeborenen Herzfehlern im Neugeborenenalter. Available online: http://www.kinderkardiologie.org/fileadmin/user_upload/Stellungnahmen/POS%20Stellungsnahme%20DGPK2%2011%2013%20final.pdf (accessed on 20 March 2018).
15. Herting, E.; Vetter, K.; Gonser, M.; Bassler, D.; Hentschel, R.; Groneck, P. Betreuung von Gesunden Reifen Neugeborenen in der Geburtsklinik. Available online: http://www.awmf.org/uploads/tx_szleitlinien/024-005l_S2k_Betreuung_von_gesunden_reifen_Neugeborenen_2012-10-abgelaufen.pdf (accessed on 20 March 2018).
16. Bärnighausen, T.; Sauerborn, R. One hundred and eighteen years of the German health insurance system: Are there any lessons for middle- and low-income countries? *Soc. Sci. Med.* **2002**, *54*, 1559–1587. [CrossRef]
17. Screening auf Kritische Angeborene Herzfehler Mittels Pulsoxymetrie bei Neugeborenen. Institut für Qualität und Wirtschaftlichkeit im Gesundheitswesen (IQWiG). Available online: https://www.iqwig.de/download/S13-01_Abschlussbericht_Pulsoxymetrie.pdf (accessed on 20 March 2018).
18. Beschluss des Gemeinsamen Bundesausschusses über eine Änderung der Richtlinie über die Früherkennung von Krankheiten bei Kindern bis zur Vollendung des 6. Lebensjahres (Kinder-Richtlinie): Screening auf Kritische Angeborene Herzfehler Mittels Pulsoxymetrie bei Neugeborenen. Available online: https://www.g-ba.de/downloads/39-261-2762/2016-11-24_Kinder-RL_Pulsoxymetrie-Screening-Neugeborene_BAnz.pdf (accessed on 20 March 2018).
19. Screening auf Kritische Angeborene Herzfehler Mittels Pulsoxymetrie bei Neugeborenen–Zusammenfassende Dokumentation. Available online: https://www.g-ba.de/downloads/40-268-4066/2016-11-24_Kinder-RL_Pulsoxymetrie-Screening-Neugeborene_ZD.pdf (accessed on 20 March 2018).
20. Kemper, A.R.; Mahle, W.T.; Martin, G.R.; Cooley, W.C.; Kumar, P.; Morrow, W.R.; Kelm, K.; Pearson, G.D.; Glidewell, J.; Grosse, S.D.; et al. Strategies for Implementing Screening for Critical Congenital Heart Disease. *Pediatrics* **2011**, *128*, e1259–e1267. [CrossRef] [PubMed]
21. Thangaratinam, S.; Brown, K.; Zamora, J.; Khan, K.S.; Ewer, A.K. Pulse oximetry screening for critical congenital heart defects in asymptomatic newborn babies: A systematic review and meta-analysis. *Lancet* **2012**, *379*, 2459–2464. [CrossRef]
22. Manzoni, P.; Martin, G.R.; Luna, M.S.; Mestrovic, J.; Simeoni, U.; Zimmermann, L.; Ewer, A.K.; Manzoni, P.; Martin, G.R.; Granelli, A.D.W.; et al. Pulse oximetry screening for critical congenital heart defects: A European consensus statement. *Lancet Child. Adolesc. Health* **2017**, *1*, 88–90. [CrossRef]

23. Narayen, I.C.; Blom, N.A.; Ewer, A.K.; Vento, M.; Manzoni, P.; te Pas, A.B. Aspects of pulse oximetry screening for critical congenital heart defects: When, how and why? *Arch. Dis. Child. Fetal Neonatal Ed.* **2016**, *101*, F162–F167. [CrossRef] [PubMed]
24. Johnson, L.C.; Lieberman, E.; O'Leary, E.; Geggel, R.L. Prenatal and newborn screening for critical congenital heart disease: Findings from a nursery. *Pediatrics* **2014**, *134*, 916–922. [CrossRef] [PubMed]
25. Quartermain, M.D.; Pasquali, S.K.; Hill, K.D.; Goldberg, D.J.; Huhta, J.C.; Jacobs, J.P.; Jacobs, M.L.; Kim, S.; Ungerleider, R.M. Variation in Prenatal Diagnosis of Congenital Heart Disease in Infants. *Pediatrics* **2015**, *136*, e378–e385. [CrossRef] [PubMed]
26. Lindinger, A.; Schwedler, G.; Hense, H.W. Prevalence of Congenital Heart Defects in Newborns in Germany: Results of the First Registration Year of the PAN Study (July 2006 to June 2007). *Klin. Padiatr.* **2010**, *222*, 321–326. [CrossRef] [PubMed]
27. Abouk, R.; Grosse, S.D.; Ailes, E.C.; Oster, M.E. Association of US State Implementation of Newborn Screening Policies for Critical Congenital Heart Disease With Early Infant Cardiac Deaths. *JAMA* **2017**, *318*, 2111–2118. [CrossRef] [PubMed]
28. Wren, C.; Reinhardt, Z.; Khawaja, K. Twenty-year trends in diagnosis of life-threatening neonatal cardiovascular malformations. *Arch. Dis. Child. Fetal Neonatal Ed.* **2008**, *93*, F33–F35. [CrossRef] [PubMed]

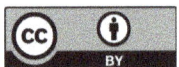 © 2018 by the authors. Licensee MDPI, Basel, Switzerland. This article is an open access article distributed under the terms and conditions of the Creative Commons Attribution (CC BY) license (http://creativecommons.org/licenses/by/4.0/).

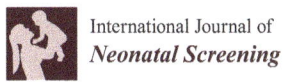

International Journal of
Neonatal Screening

Article

Critical Congenital Heart Disease Screening Using Pulse Oximetry: Achieving a National Approach to Screening, Education and Implementation in the United States

Lisa A. Wandler * and Gerard R. Martin

Children's National Heart Institute, Washington, DC 20010-2970, USA; gmartin@childrensnational.org
* Correspondence: lhom@childrensnational.org; Tel.: +01202-476-5063

Received: 19 September 2017; Accepted: 10 October 2017; Published: 19 October 2017

Abstract: A national approach to screening for critical congenital heart disease (CCHD) using pulse oximetry was undertaken in the United States. Following the scientific studies that laid the groundwork for the addition of CCHD screening to the U.S. Recommended Uniform Screening Panel (RUSP) and endorsement by professional societies, advocates including physicians, nurses, parents, medical associations, and newborn screening interest groups were able to successfully pass laws requiring the screen on a state by state basis. Public health involvement and screening requirements vary by state. However, a common algorithm, education, and implementation strategies were shared nationally as well as CCHD toolkits to aid in the implementation in hospitals. Health Resources & Services Administration (HRSA) grants to pilot states encouraged the development of a public health infrastructure around screening, data collection, and quality measures. The formation of a CCHD NewSTEPs technical advisory work group provided a systematic way to tackle challenges and share best practices by hosting monthly meetings and webinars. CCHD screening is now required in 48 states, with over 98% of U.S. births being screened for CCHD using pulse oximetry. A standard protocol has been implemented in most states. While the challenges related to screening special populations and quantifying screening outcomes through the creation of a national data repository remain; universal implementation is nearly complete.

Keywords: CCHD screening in the US; newborn screening pulse oximetry; critical congenital heart disease screening

---

1. Introduction

Critical congenital heart disease (CCHD) screening using pulse oximetry is a point of care newborn screen that relies on the detection of low blood oxygen levels to identify infants who may have CCHD or other life threatening neonatal conditions. Particularly useful for identifying asymptomatic infants with CCHD in well-baby nurseries, the importance of this screen is in its ability to allow for the detection of CCHD prior to when the infant is discharged from the birth hospital. The late detection of CCHD, after hospital discharge, has been shown to increase morbidity and mortality [1].

Congenital heart disease (CHD) is the most common birth defect. In the U.S., approximately 40,000 infants are born with CHD, with 25% of those having CCHD [2–4]. The primary targets for CCHD screening were identified through expert consensus in 2011. The list included those seven lesions most likely to be identified using pulse oximetry: hypoplastic left heart syndrome, pulmonary atresia, tetralogy of Fallot, total anomalous pulmonary venous return, transposition of the great arteries, tricuspid atresia, and truncus arteriosus [5]. This list of core conditions was expanded in 2016, this time by an expert panel convened by the Centers for Disease Control (CDC) and the

American Academy of Pediatrics (AAP) to include coarctation of the aorta, double-outlet right ventricle, Ebstein's anomaly, interrupted aortic arch, single ventricle, and other critical cyanotic lesions not specified. The expert panel also acknowledged the added benefit of identifying secondary targets, including hemoglobinopathy, hypothermia, infection (including sepsis), lung disease, noncritical CHD, persistent pulmonary hypertension, and other hypoxemic conditions as important public health targets of CCHD screening in the U.S. [6].

The goal of this article is to give an overview and insight into how the U.S. was able to achieve systematic implementation of CCHD screening using pulse oximetry including a nationally endorsed screening algorithm, centralized resources coordinated at the state and federal government levels, shared educational strategies, and toolkits; thus, moving within five years from screening in only a few hospitals, mainly associated with research studies with no state requirements, to nearly universal implementation in all but two states.

2. Early Studies and 2009 Scientific Statement

The need for additional methods to identify infants with CCHD early and prior to circulatory collapse was made very clear in one research study that investigated missed diagnosis of CCHD in California. More than 50% of CCHD deaths (up to 30 infants a year) could be attributed to late or missed diagnosis in the neonatal period in the state of California alone [7]. Evidence presented in the Chang study and others [8] demonstrated that additional methods of detection for CCHD, aside from prenatal ultrasound and physical examination of the neonate, were needed. If infants with CCHD could be identified, diagnosed, and receive an intervention (cardiovascular surgery or cardiac catheterization), survival and morbidity outcomes could be improved.

Although the concept of using pulse oximetry as a screening mechanism was explored in research articles both in the U.S. and Europe as early as 1993 [9–12], screening had not yet been implemented in U.S. newborn nurseries or required in any states. In 2005, Mississippi proposed legislation suggesting that pulse oximetry screening be used as a strategy to identify additional instances of newborns with CCHD [13]. Tennessee also considered early pulse oximetry screening legislation, but at that time, cardiologists, concerned about false positive studies, were hesitant to support the concept of CCHD screening as a state mandate [14]. Pulse oximetry screening was gaining significant attention as a potential strategy to improve the timely recognition of CCHD; the scientific community responded by reviewing the state of evidence related to the use of pulse oximetry in newborns to detect CCHD [15].

On behalf of the AAP Section on Cardiology and Cardiac Surgery, and Committee on Fetus and Newborn and the American Heart Association (AHA) Congenital Heart Defects Committee of the Council on Cardiovascular Disease in the Young, Council on Cardiovascular Nursing, and Interdisciplinary Council on Quality of Care and Outcomes Research, an expert writing group was tasked with evaluating the state of evidence on the routine use of pulse oximetry to detect CCHD. In 2009, they released a scientific statement concluding, based on an analysis of papers from 1966 to 2008, the following: CCHD was not being detected in some newborns prior to discharge from their birth hospital, resulting in significant morbidity and occasional mortality; if routine pulse oximetry is performed on asymptomatic newborns after 24 h of life but prior to discharge, additional CCHD could be detected, particularly in hospitals where on-site pediatric cardiologists and pediatric cardiovascular services were available; and that screening could be conducted at very low cost and risk of harm [15]. However, the expert group went on to emphasize that further studies in "larger populations and across a broad range of newborn delivery systems" was required to determine whether pulse oximetry testing should become the standard of care in the routine assessment of neonates [15].

3. Evidence from Europe

While the AHA/AAP expert writing group was performing their review of the evidence and grappling with the need for population level data to validate using pulse oximetry as a CCHD screening tool, researchers in Europe were poised to publish several important studies that would provide the precise evidence needed. Studies from Sweden, the United Kingdom, and Germany demonstrated that screening for CCHD at the population level had the required sensitivity and specificity to meet the criteria for newborn screening.

Perhaps most influential was a study from Sweden by Granelli et al. It was complete but not published in time to be considered in the analysis by the 2009 AAP/AHA writing group. This study analyzed 39,821 newborns who were screened using pulse oximetry and compared the strategy of physical exam alone with pulse oximetry screening alone, and in combination physical exam and pulse oximetry screening. The results were compelling, in addition to having an acceptable sensitivity (82.8% when combined with physical assessment) and specificity (97.8%); many of the false positives of pulse oximetry screening were not CCHD, but true positives for other important pathologies including persistent pulmonary hypertension of the newborn (PPHN), pneumonia, and infections, adding to the value of the screen outside of identifying unknown infants with CCHD. Although not all forms of CCHD can be detected by using pulse oximetry, this study concluded that 92% of ductal dependent cases could be identified if screening was performed in newborn delivery hospitals prior to discharge [16].

An additional study was published in 2010. It involved 34 institutions in Germany in which 42,240 infants were screened (sensitivity 77.78%, specificity 99.90%, and negative predictive value 99.99%). Based on the analysis of those screens, the study team concluded that the addition of pulse oximetry screening could substantially close the postnatal diagnostic gap (those cases of CCHD not identified through prenatal ultrasound or physical assessment) to 4.4% [17].

A meta-analysis conducted by researchers in the United Kingdom, which identified 13 high quality primary studies involving 229,421 infants screened using pulse oximetry, provided additional key support. The calculated sensitivity (76.5%) was similar to the Granelli study and the false positive rate overall was 0.14%. Interestingly, when the data was further broken down, the study found that the false positive rate, if the screening was conducted after 24 h, was significantly lower than if the screening was conducted prior to 24 h of life (false positive rate <24 h 0.5% versus >24 h 0.05%) [18]. This distinction would later factor heavily into the development of the U.S. nationally endorsed protocol. However, it may not have properly acknowledged that additional secondary conditions make up the majority of those false positives.

These studies from Europe provided valuable evidence that would help to inform the development of the U.S. recommended strategies. In fact, two of the U.S. CCHD stakeholder meetings included expert representation from among the authors of the Swedish and UK studies.

4. Call to Action as CCHD Screening Is Added to the RUSP

In October 2010, following the availability of new evidence from Europe and a formal scientific evidence review process, the Secretary's Advisory Committee on Heritable Disorders in Newborns and Children (SACHDNC), whose responsibility it is to identify, evaluate, and make recommendations on which newborn screens should be added to the Recommended Uniform Screening Panel (RUSP), evaluated the research, heard the testimony of experts and families, and agreed that CCHD screening using pulse oximetry be recommended at the national level as part of the standard of care for newborn screening in the US. An additional review to propose a plan of action and to address the evidence gaps by the Interagency Coordinating Committee (ICC) was also completed prior to endorsement by the Secretary of Health and Human Services [19].

A group of experts and stakeholders came together for a two-day meeting sponsored by SACHDNC and hosted by the American College of Cardiology (ACC) at the Heart House in January of 2011. Participants included physicians, nurses, scientists, representatives from Health Resources & Services Administration (HRSA), ACC, AAP, AHA, the American College of Medical Genetics, March of Dimes, the Association of Maternal and Child Health Programs, The Association of Public Health Laboratories (APHL), the National Institutes of Health (NIH), Centers for Disease Control and Prevention (CDC), Food and Drug Administration (FDA), parent advocacy groups, industry partners, state public health program, and healthcare organizations [19]. Initial recommendations and a screening algorithm (see Appendix A) based in large part on the Swedish protocol, specifying that screening be conducted using two limbs (the right hand and either foot) [16] were developed [5]. This algorithm was chosen mainly for its acceptable sensitivity (82.76%) and high specificity (97.88%) when paired with physical assessment. The expert group also recommended screening take place "at or around 24 h or prior to discharge" to maximize sensitivity while minimizing the number of false positives [5].

CCHD screening was added to the RUSP by Secretary Kathleen Sebelius in September of 2011 [20]. This recommendation was a first major step toward systematic implementation and represented buy-in at the federal or national level. The AAP [21], AHA, ACC, and March of Dimes also quickly endorsed CCHD screening.

The need for an additional workgroup and stakeholders meeting arose to address challenges such as the selection of screening equipment, the standards for reporting screening outcomes, the training and education of health care providers and families whose infants were being screened, payment for screening, appropriate follow-up diagnostic testing, public health involvement, and oversight and to identify areas for future research [22]. This additional work group meeting also took place at the Heart House in Washington, D.C. in February, 2012. Importantly, the recommendations from this work group included a minimum data set for both hospital level and state public health level reporting [22].

Secretary Sebelius, as a part of her 2011 adoption of CCHD screening to the RUSP, included a Federal Agency Plan of Action focused on the key areas of (1) research, (2) surveillance, (3) screening standards and infrastructure, and (4) education and training [20]. NIH was tasked with determining the impact of CCHD screening on the health outcomes of infants as well as the development of registries to help address research questions related to screening. The CDC's main area of focus would be surveillance, including the evaluation of cost-effectiveness analysis and the monitoring of CCHD mortality and its link to other health outcomes. The Health Resources and Services Administration (HRSA) was charged with completing a thorough evaluation in collaboration with SACHDNC to evaluate the potential public health impact of universal screening for CCHD and to develop screening standards, and support the development of education tools and the infrastructure required for a public health approach to this point of care screen [20].

HRSA responded by funding six CCHD state demonstration projects over a three year period, specifically to support the validation and dissemination of CCHD screening protocols and for the development of infrastructure around point-of-care screening for CCHD [23]. The state programs chosen were: Michigan, New Jersey, Utah, Virginia, Wisconsin and a consortium of five New England states (Maine, New Hampshire, Vermont, Rhode Island, and Connecticut) [23]. Shortly after the grants to the states were awarded, a third stakeholders meeting took place in Washington, D.C. in September of 2012 to kick-off and coordinate state efforts. Initial lessons learned following the completion of the grant period were published by the grantees in 2017 [23].

The need for building public health infrastructure and sharing best practices and lessons learned with other states was particularly important as CCHD screening was only the second point of care newborn screen to be implemented nationally. The first was newborn hearing screening. HRSA also provided limited funding for another CCHD specific initiative, the Newborn Screening Technical assistance and Evaluation Program (NewSTEPs). NewSTEPs partnered with federal agencies in examining CCHD screening as well as state public health newborn screening programs to provide a central platform for CCHD screening resources. It also brought together a technical assistance CCHD work group and monthly webinars specifically related to implementation, education, and the spread of CCHD best practices [24].

Since the 2011 addition to the RUSP, federal agencies continue to work towards addressing the needs identified in Secretary Sebelius' recommendations. Researchers at the CDC have published studies examining the potential impact of screening implementation on the detection of CCHD and lives saved [25], and cost-effectiveness [26].

5. State-by-State Advocacy

The addition of CCHD screening to the RUSP at the federal level is non-binding on the states. To become required by law, each state would individually need to mandate CCHD screening, which, to date, all of the states, except for three, have done, either by statute, regulation, or executive order. Indiana, New Jersey and Maryland were the first three states to require CCHD screening in 2011, prior to the addition of CCHD screening to the RUSP. Parent groups, nurses, physicians, and professional societies worked together to go state-by-state advocating that CCHD screening be adopted as law. Peak advocacy efforts within the U.S. occurred in 2013 when 25 states adopted CCHD screening [27]. By early 2015, 43 states and the District of Columbia required CCHD screening.

There are nuances in how states selected to implement, with varying levels of public health involvement. Differences in state CCHD screening laws include whether the mandate would be funded, whether all of the infants would be screened or whether exceptions to screening were permissible (special care nurseries, premature infants, out of hospital births, screening at altitude) and whether any aggregate or individual CCHD screening data would be reported. Most states choose to implement the algorithm recommended by the AAP with New Jersey, Tennessee, and Minnesota being among the few exceptions [6]. Data collection, the extent to which education was provided, and the monitoring of implementation by state public health departments also vary greatly.

By the end of 2016, only two states, Idaho and Wyoming, were not screening. One state, Kansas, implemented at all hospital newborn nurseries without a state mandate. As of September 2017, the last two states that do not require screening, Idaho and Wyoming, have proposed regulations pending that would require CCHD screening. Rapid adoption by the states can largely be contributed to the alignment of several key forces, the validation of pulse oximetry as an effective screening method at the federal level, the endorsement of screening by national professional medical societies, and the support in the form of initial financial resources by federal and state public health agencies. Parents and clinical experts also played key roles as advocates [28], testifying at both the state and federal levels in support of CCHD screening and its ability to save lives through early identification.

6. Systematic Implementation

Once required by state law, there was still considerable work to be done to implement CCHD screening in hospitals with newborn nurseries. Several different strategies were employed to ensure an efficient approach. These included the use of CCHD implementation toolkits, the sharing of educational videos for providers and families, a train-the-trainer approach, and the dissemination of resources, best practices, and solutions to common challenges through the aforementioned NewSTEPs webinars.

Systematic implementation was aided by the publication of a feasibility study conducted in Maryland, demonstrating that CCHD screening could be successfully implemented at a community hospital without the need for additional staff members, taking an average of only 3.5 min to screen and with few barriers [29]. Showing that CCHD screening was feasible in a community hospital was important. Prior to this study, most screening implementation was conducted at large, often urban centers and most often associated with research.

In 2013, NewSTEPs, which continues to function as a part of a partnership between the Association of Public Health Laboratories (APHL) and the Colorado School of Public Health, began hosting monthly CCHD technical assistance webinars to assist in the dissemination of best practices and working solutions to commonly identified challenges to screening [23]. Early topics included: educational resources available for parents and screeners, data collection including electronic reporting resources, defining roles and resources from a public health perspective, special populations, and how to address cost/equipment issues [30]. NewSTEPs, in partnership with the Pediatric Congenital Heart Association, also brought together the HRSA grantees and other leaders in CCHD for an in-person meeting in February 2014. The purpose of this meeting was to discuss the current status of CCHD screening in the U.S. and to share ideas and provide guidance for state screening programs involved in all stages of implementation [23].

Toolkits containing materials used to implement in a hospital newborn nursery made it possible to implement screening in a new hospital without having to gather and develop all of the necessary components for implementation each time. These toolkits contained important background evidence on CCHD screening, information on the screening protocol, education for providers, nurses, and parents, as well as competencies and forms to facilitate the documentation of screening results. Children's National Medical Center developed one such CCHD screening implementation toolkit that was shared nationally and adapted to be state specific in Alaska, Missouri, Utah, and Colorado. Other states, including Rhode Island, Texas, and Wisconsin also created and extensively used CCHD screening implementation toolkits within their states.

Educational videos and training modules, incorporating evidence based content, were created and shared to provide those staff tasked with implementing CCHD screening with information on the importance, benefits and limitation of screening, technical assistance in how to perform the screen as well as information for parents on understanding the screens purpose and results [31,32]. Donations from families, federal and state funds all helped support the development of these freely available resources.

7. Lessons Learned

An early concern discussed extensively in stakeholder meetings and prior to the addition to the RUSP was that CCHD screening would result in too many false positives. This initial concern was not valid; early adopters did not find that the number of false positives overwhelmed the care delivery system in the way of unnecessary referrals to specialists or unnecessary echocardiograms [33,34]. Screening with pulse oximetry is not diagnostic for CCHD, it simply identifies an infant for follow-up to determine the cause for hypoxia. Referral and assessment by a pediatric cardiologist and an echocardiogram are required for a diagnosis of CCHD. Other causes of low blood oxygen levels should also be considered, such as assessment and laboratory work for infectious or respiratory causes. This distinction was particularly important in places that were geographically isolated or remote, where an infant would have to be transported over great distances for follow-up to occur. If another cause for a failed screen could be identified first, a referral and echocardiogram may not be required. Initial U.S. recommendations for follow-up stated that a comprehensive evaluation for the causes of hypoxemia be conducted and if the hypoxemia is not explained, a diagnostic echocardiogram with interpretation by a pediatric cardiologist is needed [5]. However, subsequent research from Europe has shown that echocardiography is not always needed if another condition is found to be causing the low blood oxygen saturation, and that only 29% of those that fail the screen require echocardiograms [35]. The number of false positives in the U.S. did not result in a large number of unnecessary echocardiograms once CCHD screening implementation was underway [29,34].

Misinterpretation of the screening algorithm and protocol violations were also reported as early implementation was undertaken. These issues could be addressed or minimized by implementing quality metrics and through the use of electronic decision support tools [33,36]. Best practices are still being developed with regards to screening special populations, particularly home births, births at altitude, and evaluating whether screening of infants in neonatal intensive care units is effective [37]. Colorado requires CCHD screening of infants born at moderate altitude, accepting a higher false positive rate when compared to infants born at sea level [38]. Physicians, midwives, and nurses in Wisconsin and Pennsylvania have tailored the AAP recommended screening protocol for use in out of hospital births [30]. Best practices related to screening these special populations continue to be studied [23,24].

Although a few early adopter states have published data on their initial implementation of CCHD screening [34], states that received grants from HRSA cited the lack of sustained funding for data collection activities to be the most common and important challenge identified [23]. Initial federal and state funds were limited and not renewed. Data collection activities vary greatly by state. In some states, the public health department is not permitted to collect newborn screening data; whereas in others, such as Maryland, Minnesota, Virginia, Florida, and New Jersey results are reported centrally to the state department of health sometimes using electronic birth certificates or rely on the dried blood spot cards as the reporting mechanism. Other states have developed automated systems and have the ability to extract data directly from the pulse oximeter devices and electronically transmit and report results [23]. One survey conducted in 2015 reported that 74% of states collected CCHD screening data or had plans to do so, however, that the amount of data collected varied from aggregate results on whether infants passed or failed, to all individual screening results [27].

The dramatic variation in the amount of CCHD screening data collected and the differences in how the data is collected (electronic, paper, aggregate data vs. individual screening results) has made it difficult to analyze the data to accurately assess and inform the impact that screening has on reducing CCHD morbidity and mortality through early detection and intervention. In particular, the need for an "assessment of the certainty of diagnosis using standardized public health surveillance case definitions" is needed to be able to allow for consistent comparisons across state screening programs and over time [24]. Although a national web-based repository to collect data on CCHD screening outcomes was created through NewSTEPs, without a requirement to collect CCHD screening data, which many of the CCHD screening mandates lack, the data is not available or submitted, to date, for systematic review and analysis nationally.

8. Conclusions

During a follow-up Advisory Committee on Heritable Disorders in Newborns and Children (ACHDNC) meeting in August of 2017, committee members discussed whether CCHD screening may be one of the most successful and impactful additions to the RUSP, particularly in its ability to gain the attention and buy-in of the general public, and publicity in the form of newspaper articles and news coverage. Outcomes analysis to assess the national impact of requiring CCHD screening in the U.S. is currently underway and may rely heavily on administrative data, birth defect and death registry data in the absence of population level CCHD outcomes reporting, since no such robust U.S. clinical dataset currently exists. Data from Europe that was crucial in informing initial recommendations and strategies related to screening may continue to be informative for future U.S. algorithm refinements particularly around the question of ideal timing of the screen [39].

A preliminary report, examining state death registry data from 2007–2013, was presented to ACHDNC in the August 2017 meeting. This report focused on the impact of state policies requiring CCHD screening, and found a 33% reduction in CCHD infant deaths in those states requiring screening and a calculated potential reduction of approximately 120 infant deaths due to CCHD per year in the U.S. as a whole [40]. This reduction in infant deaths is the primary outcome hoped for by the many individuals, government entities, researchers, physicians, nurses, public health staff, industry partners, parents, and others that worked to ensure that CCHD screening using pulse oximetry would be implemented in the U.S. as a national policy. As research studies, federal and state programs continue to focus on CCHD screening, we will learn more about the granular impact of public health involvement and the implementation of screening on decreasing the late identification of infants with CCHD, and the subsequent impact on morbidity and neurodevelopmental outcomes as well as evidence based recommendations for special settings [24].

Acknowledgments: We are grateful to Lindsay Attaway for her graphic designs and editorial assistance.

Author Contributions: Lisa Wandler drafted the initial outline and first draft of the manuscript. Gerard Martin developed the conceptual framework, edited and revised the manuscript.

Conflicts of Interest: The authors declare no conflict of interest.

Appendix A

U.S. Algorithm [5]

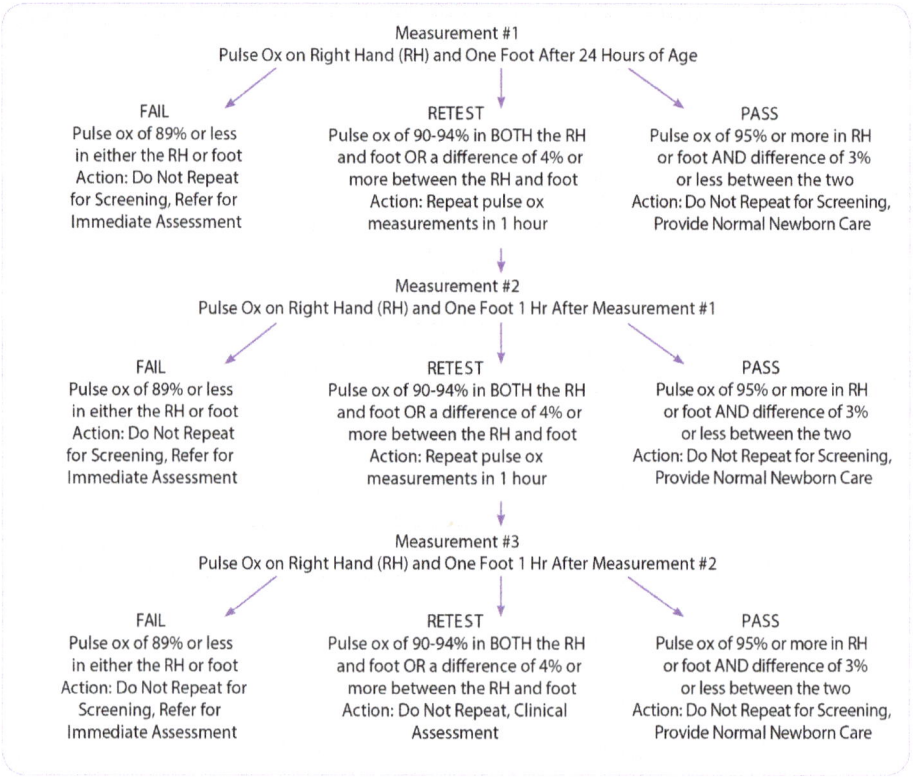

Appendix B

Timeline of U.S. Implementation

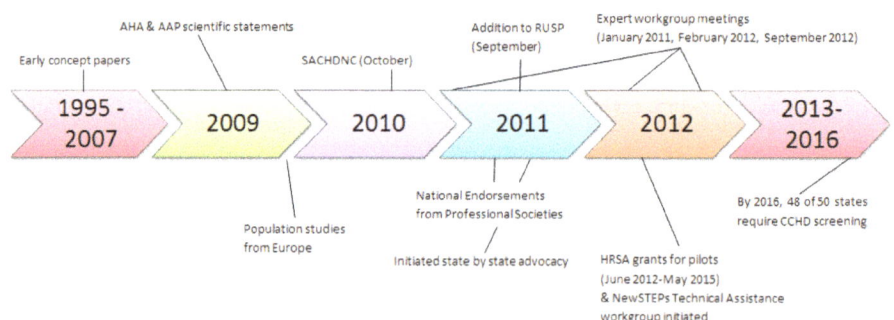

Table A1. Showing Components for Successful U.S. Implementation & Barriers Addressed.

Components for Successful Implementation	Barriers Addressed and *Solutions*
• Common algorithm/protocol for screening & follow-up • Endorsement by professional societies • Engage parents and clinical stakeholders as advocates • Federal recommendations and agency involvement • Centralized shared educational resources and dissemination of best practices/lessons learned	• Too many false positives—*In most cases, false positives are important secondary conditions* • Unnecessary referrals to pediatric cardiology and echocardiograms—*Found to be reasonable in practice* • Quality control and assurance of protocol adherence and interpretation—*Quality metrics and electronic decision support* • Screening special populations (neonatal intensive care units, at high altitude, out of hospital births)—*Best practices in development*

References

1. Eckersley, L.; Sadler, L.; Parry, E.; Finucane, K.; Gentles, T.L. Timing of diagnosis affects mortality in critical congenital heart disease. *BMJ* **2016**, *101*, 516–520. [CrossRef] [PubMed]
2. Hoffman, J.; Kaplan, S. The incidence of Congenital Heart Disease. *J. Am. Coll. Cardiol.* **2002**, *39*, 1890–1900. [CrossRef]
3. Centers for Disease Control and Prevention. Data & Statistics. Congenital Heart Defects. Available online: https://www.cdc.gov/ncbddd/heartdefects/data.html (accessed on 23 August 2017).
4. American Academy of Pediatrics. Newborn Screening for CCHD. Frequently Asked Questions. Available online: https://www.aap.org/en-us/advocacy-and-policy/aap-health-initiatives/PEHDIC/Pages/Newborn-Screening-for-CCHD.aspx (accessed on 23 August 2017).
5. Kemper, A.R.; Mahle, W.T.; Martin, G.R.; Cooley, W.C.; Kumar, P.; Morrow, W.R.; Kelm, K.; Pearson, G.D.; Glidewell, J.; Grosse, S.D.; et al. Strategies for implementing screening for critical congenital heart disease. *Pediatrics* **2011**, *128*, e1259–e1267. [CrossRef] [PubMed]
6. Oster, M.E.; Aucott, S.W.; Glidewell, J.; Hackell, J.; Kochlias, L.; Martin, G.R.; Phillippi, J.; Pinto, N.M.; Saarinen, A.; Sontag, M.; et al. Lessons Learned From Newborn Screening for Critical Congenital Heart Defects. *Pediatrics* **2016**, *137*, e20154573. [CrossRef] [PubMed]
7. Chang, R.K.; Gurvitz, M.; Rodriguez, S. Missed Diagnosis of Critical Congenital Heart Disease. *Arch. Pediatr. Adolesc. Med.* **2008**, *162*, 969–974. [CrossRef] [PubMed]
8. Mouledoux, J.H.; Walsh, W.F. Evaluating the Diagnostic Gap: Statewide Incidence of Undiagnosed Critical Congenital Heart Disease before Newborn Screening with Pulse Oximetry. *Pediatr. Cardiol.* **2013**, *34*, 1680–1686. [CrossRef] [PubMed]
9. Hoke, T.R.; Druschel, C.M.; Carter, T.; Bawa, P.K.; Mitchell, R.D.; Pathak, A.; Rowe, P.C.; Byrne, B.J. Oxygen saturation as a screening test for critical congenital heart disease: A preliminary study. *Pediatr. Cardiol.* **2002**, *23*, 403–409. [CrossRef] [PubMed]
10. Koppel, R.I.; Druschel, C.M.; Tonia, C.; Barry, E.G.; Prabhu, N.M.; Rohit, T.; Fredrick, Z.B. Effectiveness of Pulse Oximetry Screening for Congenital Heart Disease in Asymptomatic Newborns. *Pediatrics* **2003**, *111*, 45. [CrossRef]
11. Meberg, A.; Brügmann-Pieper, S.; Due, R.; Eskedal, L.; Fagerli, I.; Farstad, T.; Frøisland, D.H.; Sannes, C.H.; Johansen, O.J.; Keljalic, J.; et al. First day of life pulse oximetry screening to detect congenital heart defects. *J. Pediatr.* **2008**, *152*, 761–765. [CrossRef] [PubMed]
12. Ewer, A.K.; Middleton, L.J.; Furmston, A.T.; Bhoyar, A.; Daniels, J.P.; Thangaratinam, S.; Deeks, J.J.; Khan, K.S. Pulse oximetry screening for congenital heart defects in newborn infants (PulseOx): A test accuracy study. *Lancet* **2011**, *378*, 785–794. [CrossRef]
13. Mississippi 2005 Regular Session, House Bill 1052. 2005. Available online: http://billstatus.ls.state.ms.us/documents/2005/pdf/HB/1000-1099/HB1052IN.pdf (accessed on 11 October 2017).
14. Chang, R.K.; Rodriguez, S.; Klitzner, T.S. Screening Newborns for Congenital Heart Disease with Pulse Oximetry: Survey of Pediatric Cardiologists. *Pediatr. Cardiol.* **2009**, *30*, 20–25. [CrossRef] [PubMed]

15. Mahle, W.T.; Newburger, J.W.; Matherne, G.P.; Smith, F.C.; Hoke, T.R.; Koppel, R.; Gidding, S.S.; Beekman, R.H.; Grosse, S.D.; American Heart Association Congenital Heart Defects Committee of the Council on Cardiovascular Disease in the Young, Council on Cardiovascular Nursing, and the Interdisciplinary Council on Quality of Care and Outcomes Research. Role of Pulse Oximetry in Examining Newborns for Congenital Heart Disease: A Scientific Statement from the American Heart Association and American Academy of Pediatrics. *Circulation* **2009**, *120*, 447–458. [CrossRef] [PubMed]
16. Granelli, A.D.; Wennergren, M.; Sandberg, K.; Mellander, M.; Bejlum, C.; Inganäs, L.; Eriksson, M.; Segerdahl, N.; Agren, A.; Ekman-Joelsson, B.M.; et al. Impact of pulse oximetry screening on the detection of duct dependent congenital heart disease: A Swedish prospective screening study in 39821 newborns. *BMJ* **2009**, *338*, a3037. [CrossRef] [PubMed]
17. Riede, F.T.; Worner, C.; Dahnert, I.; Möcke, A.; Kostelka, M.; Schneider, P. Effectiveness of neonatal pulse oximetry screening for detection of critical congenital heart disease in daily clinical routine: results from a prospective multicenter study. *Eur. J. Pediatr.* **2010**, *169*, 975–981. [CrossRef] [PubMed]
18. Thangaratinam, S.; Daniels, J.; Zamora, J.; Khan, K.S.; Ewer, A.K. Pulse oximetry screening for critical congenital heart defects in asymptomatic newborn babies: a systematic review and meta-analysis. *Lancet* **2012**, *379*, 2459–2464. [CrossRef]
19. Bradshaw, E.A.; Martin, G.R. Review: Screening for critical congenital heart disease: advancing detection in the newborn. *Curr. Opin. Pediatr.* **2012**, *24*, 603–608. [CrossRef] [PubMed]
20. Sebelius, K. Secretary of Health and Human Services Recommendation for Pulse Oximetry Screening. 2011. Available online: https://www.hrsa.gov/advisorycommittees/mchbadvisory/heritabledisorders/recommendations/correspondence/cyanoticheartsecre09212011.pdf (accessed on 6 September 2017).
21. Mahle, W.T.; Martin, G.R.; Beekman, R.H.; Morrow, R.; Rosenthal, G.L.; Synder, C.S.; Minich, L.L.; Mital, S.; Towbin, J.A.; Tweddell, J.S. Endorsement of Health and Human Services Recommendation for Pulse Oximetry Screening for Critical Congenital Heart Disease Section on Cardiology and Cardiac Surgery Executive Committee. *Pediatrics* **2012**, *129*, 190–192. [CrossRef] [PubMed]
22. Martin, G.R.; Beekman, R.H.; Mikula, E.B.; Fasules, J.; Garg, L.F.; Kemper, A.R.; Morrow, W.R.; Pearson, G.D.; Mahle, W.T. Implementing Recommended Screening for Critical Congenital Heart Disease. *Pediatrics* **2013**, *132*, e185–e192. [CrossRef] [PubMed]
23. McClain, M.R.; Hokanson, J.S.; Grazel, R.; Van Naarden, B.K.; Garg, L.F.; Morris, M.R.; Moline, K.; Urquhart, K.; Nance, A.; Randall, H.; et al. Critical Congenital Heart Disease Newborn Screening Implementation: Lessons Learned. *Matern. Child. Health J.* **2017**. [CrossRef]
24. Olney, R.S.; Ailes, E.C.; Sontag, M.K. Detection of critical congenital heart defects: Review of contributions from prenatal and newborn screening. *Semin. Perinatol.* **2015**, *39*, 230–237. [CrossRef] [PubMed]
25. Peterson, C.; Ailes, E.; Riehle-Colarusso, T.; Oster, M.E.; Olney, R.S.; Cassell, C.H.; Fixler, D.E.; Carmichael, S.L.; Shaw, G.M.; Gilboa, S.M. Late detection of critical congenital heart disease among US infants: estimation of the potential impact of proposed universal screening using pulse oximetry. *JAMA Pediatr.* **2014**, *168*, 361–370. [CrossRef] [PubMed]
26. Peterson, C.; Grosse, S.D.; Oster, M.E.; Olney, R.S.; Cassell, C.H. Cost-effectiveness of routine screening for critical congenital heart disease in US newborns. *Pediatrics* **2013**, *132*, e595–e603. [CrossRef] [PubMed]
27. CDC. State Legislation, Regulations, and Hospital Guidelines for Newborn Screening for Critical Congenital Heart Defects—United States, 2011–2014. *Morb. Mort. Wkly. Rep.* **2015**, *64*, 625–630.
28. Berger, S.; Health & Science. Saving babies: An inexpensive, easy oxygen test can prevent many deaths. *The Washington Post*. 7 April 2014. Available online: https://www.washingtonpost.com/national/health-science/saving-babies-an-inexpensive-easy-oxygen-test-can-prevent-many-deaths/2014/04/07/3c6c8b2a-9b12-11e3-975d-107dfef7b668_story.html?utm_term=.dde8c8a2d734 (accessed on 23 August 2017).
29. Bradshaw, E.A.; Cuzzi, S.; Kiernan, S.; Nagel, N.; Becker, J.A.; Martin, G.R. Feasibility of implementing pulse oximetry screening for congenital heart disease in a community hospital. *J. Perinatol.* **2012**, *32*, 710–715. [CrossRef] [PubMed]
30. NewSTEPs CCHD Technical Assistance Webinars. Available online: https://newsteps.org/cchd-technical-assistance-webinars (accessed on 24 August 2017).
31. Baby's First Test, Conditions, Critical Congenital Heart Disease. Heart Smart Videos. Available online: http://www.babysfirsttest.org/newborn-screening/conditions/critical-congenital-heart-disease-cchd (accessed on 6 September 2017).

32. Newborn Screening Education. Critical Congenital Heart Disease Course sponsored by the Virginia Department of Health, The University of Virginia School of Medicine and the University of Virginia Children's Hospital. Available online: http://www.newbornscreeningeducation.org/pages/cchd (accessed on 6 September 2017).
33. Kochilas, L.K.; Lohr, J.L.; Bruhn, E.; Borman-Shoap, E.; Gams, B.L.; Pylipow, M.; Saarinen, A.; Gaviglio, A.; Thompson, T.R. Implementation of Critical Congenital Heart Disease Screening in Minnesota. *Pediatrics* **2013**, *132*, e587–e594. [CrossRef] [PubMed]
34. Garg, L.F.; Van Naarden Braun, K.; Knapp, M.M.; Anderson, T.M.; Koppel, R.I.; Hirsch, D.; Beres, L.M.; Sweatlock, J.; Olney, R.S.; Glidewell, J.; et al. Results from the New Jersey statewide critical congenital heart defects screening program. *Pediatrics* **2013**, *132*, e314–e323. [CrossRef] [PubMed]
35. Singh, A.; Rasiah, S.V.; Ewer, A.K. The impact of routine predischarge pulse oximetry screening in a regional neonatal unit. *Arch. Dis. Child. Fetal Neonatal Ed.* **2014**, *99*, F297–F302. [CrossRef] [PubMed]
36. Oster, M.E.; Kuo, K.W.; Mahle, W.T. Quality Improvement in Screening for Critical Congenital Heart Disease. *J. Pediatr.* **2014**, *164*, 67–71. [CrossRef] [PubMed]
37. Van Naarden Braun, K.; Grazel, R.; Koppel, R.; Lakshminrusimha, S.; Lohr, J.; Kumar, P.; Govindaswami, B.; Giuliano, M.; Cohen, M.; Spillane, N.; et al. Evaluation of critical congenital heart defects screening using pulse oximetry in the neonatal intensive care unit. *J. Perinatol.* **2017**, *37*, 1117–1123. [CrossRef] [PubMed]
38. Children's Hospital Colorado. Pulse Oximetry Program: Recommendations for Health Professionals. Available online: https://www.childrenscolorado.org/doctors-and-departments/departments/heart/programs-and-clinics/critical-congenital-heart-disease-screening-program/screening-toolkit-for-health-professionals/program-recommendations/ (accessed on 11 September 2017).
39. Ewer, A.K.; Martin, G.R. Newborn Pulse Oximetry Screening: Which Algorithm Is Best? *Pediatrics* **2016**, *138*, e20161206. [CrossRef] [PubMed]
40. Grosse, S. Reduction in Infant Cardiac Deaths in US States Implementing Policies to Screen Newborns for Critical Congenital Heart Disease. Available online: https://www.hrsa.gov/advisorycommittees/mchbadvisory/heritabledisorders/meetings/2017/0803/8grossecchdscreeningphimpact.pdf (accessed on 14 September 2017).

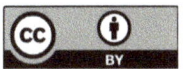

© 2017 by the authors. Licensee MDPI, Basel, Switzerland. This article is an open access article distributed under the terms and conditions of the Creative Commons Attribution (CC BY) license (http://creativecommons.org/licenses/by/4.0/).

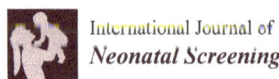 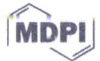

Article

A Single-Extremity Staged Approach for Critical Congenital Heart Disease Screening: Results from Tennessee

William Walsh [1,*] and Jean A. Ballweg [2]

1   Department of Pediatrics, Vanderbilt University Medical Center, Nashville, TN 37232, USA
2   Department of Pediatrics, University of Nebraska Medical Center, Nashville, TN 37232, USA; jballweg@childrensomaha.org
*   Correspondence: bill.walsh@vandbilt.edu

Received: 9 October 2017; Accepted: 14 November 2017; Published: 20 November 2017

Abstract: Tennessee initiated single-extremity staged screening by pulse oximetry for undetected CCHD in 2012. The algorithm begins with a saturation reading in the foot and allows an automatic pass if the foot pulse oximetry is 97% or greater. This was based on the principle that it is not possible to have a greater than 4% difference in the pulse oximetry between upper and lower extremities if the lower extremity is equal to or greater than 97%. This approach eliminates over 75,000 "unnecessary" pulse oximetry determinations in Tennessee each year without affecting the ability to detect CCHD before hospital discharge.

Keywords: pulse oximetry screening; screening algorithm; critical congenital heart disease; state screening; coarctation of aorta

1. Introduction

Congenital heart disease is present in approximately one in every one hundred live births in the United States. Critical congenital heart disease (CCHD) comprises a significant percentage of heart lesions. The Center for Disease Control (CDC) has identified seven congenital heart lesions that are deemed critical diseases. These seven lesions include hypoplastic left heart syndrome, pulmonary atresia, tetralogy of Fallot, total anomalous venous return, transposition of the great arteries, tricuspid atresia and truncus arteriosus.

Until pulse oximetry screening in the United States was begun, about 30% of infants with CCHD—or 6 per 10,000 babies—with the seven critical congenital heart disease lesions identified by the CDC were not diagnosed until after initial hospital discharge [1].

With the recommendation for screening in 2011, the USA Secretary of Health and Human Services recommended routine newborn pulse oximetry screening be performed prior to hospital discharge. As of 2015, 46 states and the District of Columbia require hospitals to screen newborns for critical CCHDs [2].

The protocol recommended by the AHA and CDC for screening was based on extensive review of evidence from major European trials [3–6].

In 2011, the AHA and the CDC decided upon a protocol that evaluates the pulse oximetry reading of the infant on a hand and foot after 24 h of age. To avoid the problem of multiple false positives, it was decided to repeat the screen twice prior to declaring the infant a failure [7].

Seven key lesions which would be expected to have a low saturation were targeted by the AHA and comprise the group of lesions referred to as CCHD as defined above. In addition to the 7 identified CCHDs, the CDC has targeted an additional five lesions when studying CCHD screening.

These five lesions include coarctation of the aorta, double outlet right ventricle, Ebstein's anomaly, interrupted aortic arch and single ventricle lesions other than HLHS.

This protocol for screening two extremities was based on the possibility that a baby with secondary targets such as coarctation may have decreased saturations in the lower extremity compared to the upper, and therefore a persistent difference greater than 3% between upper and lower extremity was considered an indication for further evaluation. Using this protocol, it was estimated that about half the infants with CCHD who would have been missed by lack of prenatal diagnosis and absence of signs in the newborn nursery would be identified by a failed pulse oximetry screening test [8].

It was estimated that, each year, about 875 more newborns with a CCHD could be identified at birth hospitals using pulse oximetry newborn screening, but an equal number (880 babies) might still be missed each year in the United States. Lesions that were of concern for being missed and significant included truncus arteriosus, coarctation of the aorta and interrupted aortic arch.

The state of Tennessee had been evaluating the possibility of screening since 2006 [9]. We and the state reported on the incidence of missed CCHD, and identified that a diagnostic gap existed in Tennessee prior to the beginning of state-wide screening [10].

Based on our experience and the literature, it was estimated that pulse oximetry would detect CCHD in 5 to 7 Tennessee infants who would otherwise be missed. It was also suggested that the upper extremity pulse oximetry reading would be unnecessary if an initial foot pulse oximetry reading was 97% or higher, since it would be impossible to have a difference of greater than 3%. Therefore, the Genetics Advisory Committee of the state of Tennessee presented to the Commissioner of Health a modified Tennessee algorithm with an initial assessment of a single lower extremity reading, which, if 97% or higher a second, upper extremity, test was not required. Figure 1 The two-year results of this screening algorithm are presented in this report.

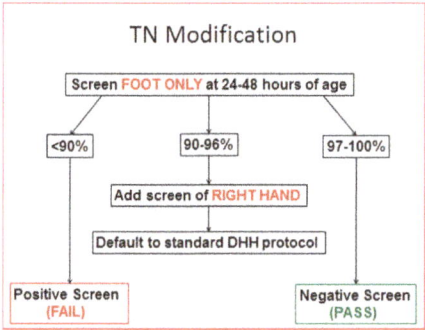

Figure 1. Foot only screen, if the pulse oximetry level is 97% or higher, the test is a pass and no upper extremity result is obtained, if the level is less than 90% the infant fails and is referred for further evaluation. A measurement of 90–96% results in a default to the AHA, CDC algorithm.

2. Materials and Methods

The State of Tennessee Health Department collected data on pulse oximetry screening as part of the State Genetics screening program on all live births. The State established a separate CCHD screening task force to monitor and assess newborn pulse oximetry screening. The pulse oximetry data are gathered from the pulse oximetry screening form on each metabolic screening blood spot test.

Surveillance for missed cases of CCHD was done through reports from the separate State of Tennessee Birth Defects Registry and the TIPQC missed-CCHD database as previously reported [10].

De-identified information collected by the TIPQC registry of missed cases included the neonate's diagnosis, age at diagnosis, presenting symptoms, and outcome. For the purpose of the registry, CCHD was defined as severe and life-threatening CHD requiring either surgical or catheter-based intervention in the first month of life. Reportable lesions included the 12 CDC targeted lesion which were ductal dependent lesions and lesions resulting in hypoxia. Acyanotic and non-ductal-dependent congenital heart defects requiring semi-elective surgical repair (tetralogy of Fallot without cyanosis, atrioventricular septal defect, atrial septal defect, ventricular septal defect, and patent ductus arteriosus) were excluded from the study.

3. Results

In 2013, there were 84,964 births, and in 2014 there were 87,184 births, for a total of 172,148 births in 2013–2014. During that time 95% (163,699) submitted pulse oximetry screening data. From that cohort, 96% passed with foot only evaluations. This eliminated the need for a second pulse oximetry reading in 156,948 infants.

For these 2 years, 232 infants failed the screen, with 51 true positives, or 22%. Eight babies had no prenatal suspicion or clinical signs, and were picked up solely by the screening tool. During the same period, there were 13 infants with CCHD not picked up by the screen. Ten of these had left-sided obstruction, which subsequently presented with clinical signs between day of life 3 and 30. Two infants were found to have TAPVR, one of whom was found on autopsy review after unexplained death at 14 days of age. One baby with no recorded screen presented with Tetralogy of Fallot and one with coactation presented at 9 days of age.

4. Discussion

Pulse oximetry screening for CCHD is a valuable adjunct to physical exam and clearly worth the effort. Even in the false positive cases, there are a significant number of infants with other disorders who benefit from evaluation and treatment. We did not systematically track all the babies who failed and who did not have CCHD, but we found a case of intracranial hemorrhage with apnea, a nasal lacrimal tumor, several babies with pneumonia and sepsis. It is clear that no baby should be discharged with a saturation of less than 95% without a clinical diagnosis [11].

The Tennessee algorithm saved 150,000 unnecessary pulse oximetry readings and still detected the predicted number of CCHD cases.

Using the cost data from Peterson et al. [12], and assuming the pulse oximeter probe is not changed between sites, the time necessary for screening would be reduced from 9 to 5 min; based on the Peterson approximation of average hourly nursing salary, the labor cost would be reduced from $6.68 to $3.71 per screen; it would therefore cost approximately $3.00 per baby, or over $240,000 per year, in Tennessee to obtain a pulse oximetry reading in the upper extremity, which could not be more than 3% greater than the foot reading. In addition to this financial cost, nursing time is valuable and better-used counseling families on newborn care, including Safe Sleep teaching or feeding.

In discussion with physician heath care leaders in other states, the major objection to using the Tennessee approach is the lack of endorsement by the CDC, and the concern that it is "too complicated". However, in discussion with nursing leaders, it is almost instantaneously understood that if the foot saturation is 97% or higher, it is not possible for the hand to be over 3% higher, and thus an upper extremity saturation is unnecessary. Thangaratinam et al., in their meta-analysis [13], actually showed no benefit from additional two-extremity testing. However, it is clear from the data reported that, although they are rare, babies with a true differences in saturation due to right to left ductal shunting can be identified, and the two-extremity test should be used whenever there is a possibility of an abnormal result. In the future, new technology may also allow two-site pulse oximetry to detect coarctation of the aorta by using pulsatility information [14].

The possibility of a reversal of saturations due to a TGA is not uncommon, but this condition would also have to be associated with a saturation of over 97% in the foot. To date, there have been no actual reports of such a condition. To require an additional 150,000 pulse oximetry readings each year looking for such a rare condition would not be cost-effective.

The 13 babies over two years with false negative results are particularly concerning. It is difficult to identify false negative cases, and we were fortunate in developing a state-wide voluntary reporting system. No screen result was found on 2 infants, one baby with Tetralogy had no screen recorded, and was found to be a home birth without pulse oximetry available. The other baby with coarctation presented at 9 days, and had no screen reported; this was during the first month of establishing the screening program. We have subsequently worked with our mid-wives in TN, and all have portable pulse oximetry capability and education. In addition, through the state genetics quality improvement program, there is now documented screening on over 97% of all infants. Tennessee does not require the actual saturation levels to be reported, just pass or fail, and whether one or two extremities were tested. The 11 false negatives that were screened passed with a single lower extremity test of over 97%. Nine of these infants were left-sided obstructed lesions, and upon final presentation had saturations ranging from 92 to 100%. There was one TAPVR who presented with respiratory distress, and there was one death of a baby with TAPVR who presented at 2 weeks of age in arrest; both had passed the screen. Without prospective saturation data, it is not possible to know whether some of these babies would have been diagnosed by the CDC algorithm.

Extrapolating the savings from using the Tennessee approach nationwide would result in 3.8 million fewer pulse oximetry tests, representing approximately $10 million dollars in savings without a loss of screening efficacy [12].

A major drawback to a staged single-extremity initial oximetry testing is the need for reeducation and recreation of the multiple, already existent, excellent educational programs in place in many states. CDC and AHA policy makers may decide that such effort may not be worth the benefit. Certainly, for those states that have not yet established a pulse oximetry screening program, using the most efficient approach would be beneficial.

5. Conclusions

The Tennessee single extremity algorithm can more efficiently detect infants with CCHD and should be considered by new screening programs.

Author Contributions: William Walsh Conceived of the single extremity pulse oximetry algorithm, organized the State of Tennessee to use it, created the TIPQC task force and reviewed all the collected data and wrote this report. Jean A. Ballweg Detected and reviewed missed cases, provided feedback to the state CCHD detection committee and reviewed and edited this article.

Conflicts of Interest: The authors declare no conflict of interest.

Abbreviations

AAP	Academy of Pediatrics
AHA	American Heart Association
CHD	Congenital heart disease
CCHD	Critical congenital heart disease
CI	Confidence interval
CoA	Coarctation of the aorta
TIPQC	Tennessee Initiative for Perinatal Quality Care
TN	Tennessee

References

1. Wren, C.; Reinhardt, Z.; Khawaja, K. Twenty-year trends in diagnosis of life-threatening neonatal cardiovascular malformations. *Arch. Dis. Child.* **2008**, *93*, F33–F35. [CrossRef] [PubMed]
2. Oster, M.E.; Aucott, S.W.; Gildewell, J.; Hackell, J.; Kohilas, L.; Martin, G.R.; Phillippi, J.; Pinto, N.M.; Saarinen, A.; Sontag, M.; et al. Lessons Learned From Newborn Screening for Critical Congenital Heart Defects. *Pediatrics* **2016**, *137*, e20154573. [CrossRef] [PubMed]

3. Riede, F.T.; Worner, C.; Dahnert, I.; Mockel, A.; Kostelka, M.; Schneider, P. Effectiveness of neonatal pulse oximetry screening for detection of critical congenital heart disease in daily clinical routine—Results from a prospective multicenter study. *Eur. J. Pediatr.* **2010**, *169*, 975–981. [CrossRef] [PubMed]
4. De-Wahl Granelli, A.; Wennergren, M.; Sandberg, K.; Mellander, M.; Bejum, C.; Inganas, L.; Eriksson, M.; Segerdahl, N.; Ågren, A.; Ekman-Joelsson, B.-M.; et al. Impact of pulse oximetry screening on the detection of duct dependent congenital heart disease: A Swedish prospective screening study in 39,821 newborns. *BMJ* **2009**, *338*, a3037. [CrossRef] [PubMed]
5. Ewer, A.K.; Middleton, L.J.; Furmston, A.T.; Bhoyar, A.; Daniels, J.P.; Thangaratinam, S.; Deeks, J.J.; Khan, K.S.; PulseOx Study Group. Pulse oximetry screening for congenital heart defects in newborn infants (PulseOx): A test accuracy study. *Lancet* **2011**, *378*, 785–794. [CrossRef]
6. Thangaratinam, S.; Daniels, J.; Ewer, A.K.; Zamora, J.; Khan, K.S. Accuracy of pulse oximetry in screening for congenital heart disease in asymptomatic newborns: A systematic review. *Arch. Dis. Child.* **2007**, *92*, F176–F180. [CrossRef] [PubMed]
7. Kemper, A.R.; Mahle, W.T.; Martin, G.R.; Cooley, W.C.; Kumar, P.; Morrow, W.R.; Kelm, K.; Pearson, G.D.; Glidewell, J.; Grosse, S.D.; et al. Strategies for Implementing Screening for Critical Congenital Heart Disease. *Pediatrics* **2011**, *128*, e1259–e1267. [CrossRef] [PubMed]
8. Ailes, E.C.; Gilboa, S.M.; Honein, M.A.; Oster, M.E. Estimated Number of Infants Detected and Missed by Critical Congenital Heart Defect Screening. *Pediatrics* **2015**, *135*, 1001–1012. [CrossRef] [PubMed]
9. Liske, M.R.; Greeley, C.S.; Law, D.J.; Reich, J.D.; Morrow, W.R.; Baldwin, H.S.; Graham, T.P.; Strauss, A.W.; Kavanaugh-McHugh, A.L.; Walsh, W.F. Report of the Tennessee Task Force on Screening Newborn Infants for Critical Congenital Heart Disease. *Pediatrics* **2006**, *118*, 1250–1256. [CrossRef] [PubMed]
10. Mouledoux, J.H.; Walsh, W.F. Evaluating the Diagnostic Gap: Statewide Incidence of Undiagnosed Critical Congenital Heart Disease before Newborn Screening with Pulse Oximetry. *Pediatr. Cardiol.* **2013**, *34*, 1680–1686. [CrossRef] [PubMed]
11. Ewer, A.K.; Furnston, A.T.; Middleton, L.J.; Deeks, J.J.; Daniels, J.P.; Pattison, H.M.; Powell, R.; Roberts, T.E.; Barton, P.; Auguste, P.; et al. Pulse oximetry as a screening test for congenital heart defects in newborn infants: A test accuracy study with evaluation of acceptability and cost-effectiveness. *Health Technol. Assess.* **2012**, *16*, 1–184.
12. Peterson, C.; Grosse, S.D.; Oster, M.E.; Olney, R.S.; Cassell, C.H. Cost-effectiveness of routine screening for critical congenital heart disease in US newborns. *Pediatrics* **2013**, *132*, e595–e603. [CrossRef] [PubMed]
13. Thangaratinam, S.; Brown, K.; Zamora, J.; Khan, K.S.; Ewer, A.K. Pulse oximetry screening for critical congenital heart defects in asymptomatic newborn babies: A systematic review and meta-analysis. *Lancet* **2012**, *379*, 2459–2464. [CrossRef]
14. Granelli, A.W.; Ostman-Smith, I. Noninvasive peripheral perfusion index as a possible tool for screening for critical left heart obstruction. *Acta Paediatr.* **2007**, *96*, 1455–1459. [CrossRef] [PubMed]

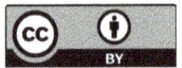

© 2017 by the authors. Licensee MDPI, Basel, Switzerland. This article is an open access article distributed under the terms and conditions of the Creative Commons Attribution (CC BY) license (http://creativecommons.org/licenses/by/4.0/).

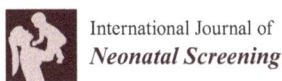

International Journal of
Neonatal Screening

Article

Congenital Critical Heart Defect Screening in a Health Area of the Community of Valencia (Spain): A Prospective Observational Study

Elena Cubells [1], Begoña Torres [2], Antonio Nuñez-Ramiro [1], Manuel Sánchez-Luna [3], Isabel Izquierdo [1] and Máximo Vento [1,2,*]

[1] Division of Neonatology, Hospital Universitario y Politécnico La Fe, 46026 Valencia, Spain; cubecha@hotmail.com (E.C.); aguillermo9nr@hotmail.com (A.N.-R.); izquierdo_isamac@gva.es (I.I.)
[2] Instituto de Investigación Sanitaria La Fe, 46026 Valencia, Spain; bego.torresg@gmail.com
[3] Division of Neonatology, Hospital Universitario Gregorio Marañón, 28007 Madrid, Spain; msluna@salud.madrid.org
* Correspondence: maximo.vento@uv.es or vento_max@gva.es; Tel.: +34-96-124-5688 (ext. 5686)

Received: 9 November 2017; Accepted: 2 January 2018; Published: 5 January 2018

Abstract: Despite the progress in the fetal echocardiographic detection of congenital critical heart defects and neonatal physical examination, a significant number of newborn infants are discharged and readmitted to the hospital in severe condition due to cardiac failure or collapse. The aim of this study was to assess the incidence of undetected critical congenital heart disease (CCHD) by a pulse oximetry-screening program in the maternity wards of hospitals with Perinatal Services in a specific geographic area. This is a prospective observational study performed in in the health area corresponding to the city of Valencia. Eligible infants were consecutively admitted newborn infants in the maternities of the participating hospitals with negative fetal echocardiography after normal physical examination in the delivery room. All patients were screened following a specific pulse oximetry protocol before discharge. A total of 8856 newborn infants were screened. A total of three babies presented with severe congenital cardiac malformation and two babies presented with early onset sepsis. Sensitivity was 100% and specificity was 99.97%, with a positive predictive value of 60% and negative predictive value of 100%. Pulse oximetry screening programs in the early neonatal period constitute a valuable tool to avoid inadvertent hospital discharge of severe cardiac malformations and the subsequent life-threatening complications derived.

Keywords: oxygen saturation; pulse oximetry; critical congenital heart disease; screening; newborn

1. Introduction

Congenital critical heart defects (CCHD), defined as those needing invasive medical intervention or those that can produce death within the first 30 days after delivery [1], may in many cases exhibit signs and symptoms that develop after hospital discharge, potentially resulting in collapse and death. Today, prenatal fetal heart ultrasound can detect many such cases, but still some of them can be missed [2]. In addition, both physical examination of the neonate after birth can further detect congenital cardiac malformations, but not all are found [3,4]. Moreover, low oxygen saturation can also be missed clinically [5,6]. Under these circumstances, pulse oximetry appears to be a reliable screening technique in neonates before hospital discharge. It is simple, noninvasive, low-cost, and very reliable in the detection of hypoxemia, and therefore has been recommended as a screening tool [7,8]. Upon adding neonatal pulse oximetry screening to prenatal ultrasound detection and postnatal clinical exam, the diagnosis rate of CCHD increases [9] and thus the undiagnosed cases of CCHD are reduced to less than 10% of total CCHD [10].

In September 2011, the US Health and Human Services (HHS) Secretary's Advisory Committee on Heritable Disorders in Newborns and Children recommended that critical congenital heart diseases (CCHD) to be added to the neonatal screening panel based on the evidence of a large number of newborns screened in Sweden and England [11–13].

In a large meta-analysis in 2012, 13 eligible studies with data for 229,421 newborn babies were analyzed. Pulse oximetry was demonstrated to be highly specific for the detection of critical congenital heart defects with moderate sensitivity [14]. More recently, in a Chinese multicenter study, 122,738 consecutive newborn babies (120,707 asymptomatic and 2031 symptomatic) were screened, detecting congenital heart disease in 1071 (157 critical and 330 major) [15].

We aimed to assess the relevance of universal screening for critical congenital heart disease (CCHD) in a specific health area (Valencia, Spain) where fetal detection of cardiac malformations by echocardiography had been substantially implemented in recent years.

2. Population and Methods

This is a prospective observational pilot study performed in the health area of Valencia (Spain). The study protocol was approved by the Internal Review Board (IRB) of the Hospital Universitario y Politécnico La Fe (Valencia, Spain). Parents/guardians of all recruited patients gave informed consent. A total of 12 hospitals, including level I (rural hospital, n = 5), level II (medium sized city hospital, n = 5), and level III hospitals [2], were included for a 6-month period. Eligible infants were newborn babies admitted to the maternity wards with normal fetal ultrasound evaluation for CCDH and normal newborn examination by a neonatologist in the delivery room. Babies with suspicious fetal echocardiography or abnormalities in the physical examination (color, murmurs, pulse abnormalities) were evaluated by a pediatric cardiologist and disregarded for the study.

Included patients were screened between 24–48 h after birth, following the protocol shown in Figure 1. Newborn infants with a positive or doubtful screening were admitted to the Neonatal Intensive Care Unit (NICU) where the clinical, analytical, and echocardiographic study was completed by neonatologists and pediatric cardiologists. After reaching a diagnosis, babies remained in the NICU for treatment or were discharged home.

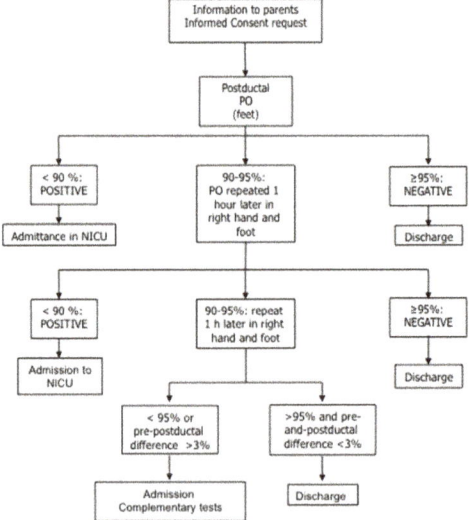

Figure 1. Flow diagram describing the protocol of the Pulsimat study for the screening of critical congenital heart disease. PO: pulse oximetry.

3. Results

Figure 2 shows the flow diagram of the study. From a total of 11,531 newborn infants born in the participating hospitals, 66 babies were diagnosed with CCHD, representing 5.8 per thousand newborn infants. Out of these, 36 patients had CCHD detected in utero and confirmed at birth (3.1 per 1000 births), 27 were diagnosed after birth based on clinical symptoms and echocardiography (2.3 per 1000 births), and three were detected by pulse oximetry screening at discharge (0.26 per thousand live births). A total of 8856 representing 78.6% of all births were screened for critical CCHD. Out of these, five had a positive pulse oximetry screen. However, two cases were caused by respiratory distress secondary to early onset sepsis; thus, only the remaining three cases were due to CCDH, specifically, total anomalous venous return.

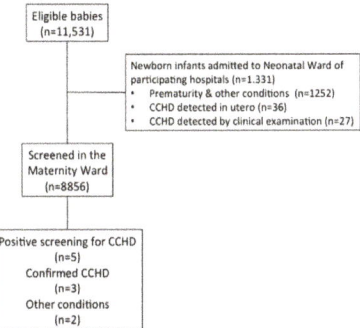

Figure 2. Consort diagram describing eligible patients, disregarded, and finally screened for critical congenital heart disease (CCHD) in the Pulsimat study.

Hence, in the 6-month study period, a total of 66 babies were diagnosed with CCHD; 36 in utero (54.5%), 27 (41.6%) ex utero by clinical examination, and three by pulse oximetry screening at discharge, representing 4.5% of the total instances of CCHD.

Table 1 shows the values for sensitivity, specificity, positive predictive value, and negative predictive value.

Table 1. Screening for congenital cardiac heart defects: analysis of results.

Pulse oximetry	Echocardiography		
	Positive	Negative	Total
Positive	3	2	5
Negative	0	8851	8851
Total	3	8853	8856

4. Discussion

It has been estimated that 30% of all CCHD patients have a late diagnosis and could benefit from neonatal screening [16]. As most previous studies demonstrated that non-cardiac conditions could also be detected by pulse oximetry, false positive detection can represent another advantage of the screening [13,17]. In our study, the detection of CCHD in utero (fetal echocardiography) plus ex utero after clinical examination represented 95.5% of the total, while 4.5% of the babies with CCHD were detected by pre-discharge screening. Interestingly, two patients that would have been discharged home with early onset sepsis had a positive screening and were admitted to the NICU. In June 2013, an international group of neonatologists and cardiologists met in Torino (Italy) with the chief investigators from two European screening studies of pulse oximetry to discuss strategies to develop Europe-wide recommendations for CCHD screening. They concluded that there is a need for a European Consensus on CCDH screening in Europe [18]. Recently, a panel from The European Pulse Oximetry Screening Workgroup investigating pulse oximetry screening for critical congenital heart defects published a European consensus statement that recommended the use of pulse oximetry for the early detection of CCDH in all European countries, using new-generation equipment that is motion tolerant; screening after 6 h of delivery and before discharge from the birth center, preferably within the 24 h after birth; and using two extremities, the right hand and either foot [19]. In addition, guidelines for the management of CCDH have been implemented, including practical aspects and nomograms to facilitate the management of these babies [20]. Finally, the Committee on Standards of the Spanish Neonatal Society (SENeo) has very recently published the National Guidelines for the Screening of Critical Congenital Heart Defects [21]. SENeo recommends performing the screening at >24 h after birth; however, each center should analyze its owns circumstances; in some centers performing screening at <12 h after birth could be preferable, despite the increase in false positives. If express discharge is performed, then any time after birth is recommended. It is also recommended to perform pre- and post-ductal pulse oximetry with motion tolerant devices that are also reliable at low saturations. The ranges of normality are similar to those defined by the European Consensus, with an absolute positivity with SpO2 values <90% and negativity with values ≥95% in any extremity, and a difference ≥3% between pre- and post-ductal pulses. In this scenario, we encourage every European country to implement the guideline that best suits their health organization and characteristics of the population.

Our study has obvious limitations. The number of patients and the geographical area are both small, and thus do not represent the entire Valencian community with 55,000 deliveries per year. However, it reveals that despite the excellent prenatal and postnatal detection of CCHD, approximately 5% of these babies would have been discharged home from the hospital. We could speculate that if we translate these numbers to the entire population of our community, at least 15 newborn infants could have been discharged yearly with a life-threatening condition, although the data obtained in our study do not support this conclusion. We did not see any false negative cases, although they have been described in other studies. Unluckily, the number of patients included in our study was relatively small and hindered the possibility of detecting such cases. In addition, our study revealed that it is feasible to systematically perform pulse oximetry screening in the maternity ward without implying a relevant additional workload for the nursing staff. Finally, it is worth mentioning that pulse oximetry screening can also promptly detect other severe conditions, such as early onset sepsis, that went undiagnosed in the routine clinical examination. The Spanish Neonatal Society (SENeo) is very soon going to put forward a protocol for the screening of CCHD that will be adopted by all the maternity wards in our country [21].

Author Contributions: Elena Cubells, Begoña Torres, Antonio-Nuñez Ramiro recruited the patients, introduced the data in the electronic registry, and performed the statistics. Manuel Sánchez-Luna, Isabel Izquierdo and Maximo Vento conceived the study, designed the study protocol and drafted and approved the final version of the manuscript.

Conflicts of Interest: The authors declare no conflict of interest.

References

1. Schultz, A.H.; Localio, A.R.; Clark, B.J.; Ravishankar, C.; Videon, N.; Kimmel, S.E. Epidemiologic features of the presentation of critical congenital heart disease: Implications for screening. *Pediatrics* **2008**, *121*, 751–757. [CrossRef] [PubMed]
2. Liu, H.; Zhou, J.; Feng, Q.L.; Gu, H.T.; Wan, G.; Zhang, H.M.; Xie, Y.J.; Li, X.S. Fetal echocardiography for congenital heart disease diagnosis: A meta-analysis, power analysis and missing data analysis. *Eur. J. Prev. Cardiol.* **2015**, *22*, 1531–1547. [CrossRef] [PubMed]

3. Górska-Kot, A.; Błaz, W.; Pszeniczna, E.; Rusin, J.; Materna-Kiryluk, A.; Homa, E.; Hejda, G.; Franus, J. Trends in diagnosis and prevalence of critical congenital heart defects in the Podkarpacie province in 2002–2004, based on data from the Polish Registry of Congenital Malformations. *J. Appl. Genet.* **2006**, *47*, 191–194. [CrossRef] [PubMed]
4. Meberg, A.; Andreassen, A.; Brunvand, L.; Markestad, T.; Moster, D.; Nietsch, L.; Silberg, I.E.; Skålevik, J.E. Pulse oximetry screening as a complementary strategy to detect critical congenital heart defects. *Acta Paediatr.* **2009**, *98*, 682–686. [CrossRef] [PubMed]
5. Hoffman, J.I. It is time for routine neonatal screening by pulse oximetry. *Neonatology* **2011**, *99*, 1–9. [CrossRef] [PubMed]
6. O'Donnell, C.P.; Kamlin, C.O.; Davis, P.G.; Carlin, J.B.; Morley, C.J. Clinical assessment of infant colour at delivery. *Arch. Dis. Child. Fetal Neonatal Ed.* **2007**, *92*, F465–F467. [CrossRef] [PubMed]
7. Mikrou, P.; Singh, A.; Ewer, A.K. Pulse oximetery screening for critical congenital heart defects: A repeat UK national survey. *Arch Dis. Child. Fetal Neonatal. Ed.* **2017**, *10*, F558–F559.
8. Mahle, W.T.; Martin, G.R.; Beekman, R.H., III; Morrow, W.R. Section on Cardiology and Cardiac Surgery Executive Committee. Endorsement of Health and Human Services recommendation for pulse oximetry screening for critical congenital heart disease. *Pediatrics* **2012**, *129*, 190–192. [PubMed]
9. Riede, F.T.; Wörner, C.; Dähnert, I.; Möckel, A.; Kostelka, M.; Schneider, P. Effectiveness of neonatal pulse oximetry screening for detection of critical congenital heart disease in daily clinical routine—Results from a prospective multicenter study. *Eur. J. Pediatr.* **2010**, *169*, 975–981. [CrossRef] [PubMed]
10. Ewer, A.K. Pulse oximetry screening: Do we have enough evidence now? *Lancet* **2014**, *384*, 725–726. [CrossRef]
11. Sebelius, K. *Secretary of Health and Human Services Recommendation for Pulse Oximetry Screening*; Department of Health and Human Services: Washington, DC, USA, 2011. Available online: http://www.hrsa.gov/advisorycommittees/mchbadvisory/heritabledisorders/recommendations/correspondence/cyanoticheartsecre09212011.pdf (accessed on 27 November 2017).
12. De-Wahl Granelli, A.; Wennergren, M.; Sandberg, K.; Mellander, M.; Bejlum, C.; Inganäs, L.; Eriksson, M.; Segerdahl, N.; Agren, A.; Ekman-Joelsson, B.M.; et al. Impact of pulse oximetry screening on the detection of duct dependent congenital heart disease: A Swedish prospective screening study in 39,821 newborns. *BMJ* **2009**, *338*, a3037. [CrossRef] [PubMed]
13. Ewer, A.K.; Middleton, L.J.; Furmston, A.T.; Bhoyar, A.; Daniels, J.P.; Thangaratinam, S.; Deeks, J.J.; Khan, K.S.; PulseOx Study Group. Pulse oximetry screening for congenital heart defects in newborn infants (PulseOx): A test accuracy study. *Lancet* **2011**, *378*, 785–794. [CrossRef]
14. Thangaratinam, S.; Brown, K.; Zamora, J.; Khan, K.S.; Ewer, A.K. Pulse oximetry screening for critical congenital heart defects in asymptomatic newborn babies: A systematic review and meta-analysis. *Lancet* **2012**, *379*, 2459–2464. [CrossRef]
15. Zhao, Q.M.; Ma, X.J.; Ge, X.L.; Liu, F.; Yan, W.L.; Wu, L.; Ye, M.; Zhang, J.; Gao, Y.; Jia, B.; et al. Pulse oximetry with clinical assessment to screen for congenital heart disease in neonates in China: A prospective study. *Lancet* **2014**, *384*, 747–754. [CrossRef]
16. Peterson, C.; Ailes, E.; Riehle-Colarusso, T.; Oster, M.E.; Olney, R.S.; Cassell, C.H.; Fixler, D.E.; Carmichael, S.L.; Shaw, G.M.; Gilboa, S.M.; et al. Late detection of critical congenital heart disease among US infants: Estimation of the potential impact of proposed universal screening using pulse oximetry. *JAMA Pediatr.* **2014**, *168*, 361–370. [CrossRef] [PubMed]
17. De-Wahl Granelli, A.; Meberg, A.; Ojala, T.; Steensberg, J.; Oskarsson, G.; Mellander, M. Nordic pulse oximetry screening—Implementation status and proposal for uniform guidelines. *Acta Paediatr.* **2014**, *103*, 1136–1142. [CrossRef] [PubMed]
18. Ewer, A.K.; Granelli, A.D.; Manzoni, P.; Sánchez Luna, M.; Martin, G.R. Pulse oximetry screening for congenital heart defects. *Lancet* **2013**, *382*, 856–857. [CrossRef]
19. Manzoni, P.; Martin, G.R.; Luna, M.S.; Mestrovic, J.; Simeoni, U.; Zimmermann, L.; Ewer, A.K. Pulse oximetry screening for critical congenital heart defects: a European consensus statement. *Lancet Child Adolesc. Health* **2017**, *1*, 88–90. [CrossRef]

20. Haas, N.A.; Franke, J. Mangement of a child with cyanosis. Guidelines for the management of congenital heart disease. *Cardiol. Young* **2017**, *27* (Suppl. 3), S3–S4.
21. Sánchez Luna, M.; Pérez Muñuzuri, A.; Sanz López, E.; Leante Castellanos, J.L.; Benavente Fernández, I.; Ruiz Campillo, C.W.; Sánchez Redondo, M.D.; Vento Torres, M.; Rite Gracia, S. Pulse oximetry screening of critical congenital heart defects in the neonatal period. The Spanish National Neonatal Society recommendation. *An. Pediatr.* **2017**. [CrossRef]

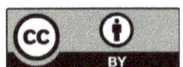

© 2018 by the authors. Licensee MDPI, Basel, Switzerland. This article is an open access article distributed under the terms and conditions of the Creative Commons Attribution (CC BY) license (http://creativecommons.org/licenses/by/4.0/).

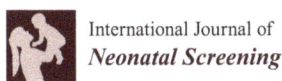

Early Detection with Pulse Oximetry of Hypoxemic Neonatal Conditions. Development of the IX Clinical Consensus Statement of the Ibero-American Society of Neonatology (SIBEN)

Augusto Sola [1] and Sergio G. Golombek [2,3,*]

[1] Professor of Pediatrics and Neonatology, Medical Executive Director of SIBEN, Wellington, FL 33414, USA; augusto.sola@siben.net
[2] President of SIBEN, Professor of Pediatrics and Clinical Public Health, New York Medical College, 40 Sunshine Cottage RD, Valhalla, NY 10595, USA
[3] Attending Neonatologist, Maria Fareri Children's Hospital at Westchester Medical Center, 100 Woods Road, Valhalla, NY 10595, USA
* Correspondence: sergio_golombek@nymc.edu

Received: 2 October 2017; Accepted: 11 February 2018; Published: 1 March 2018

Abstract: This article reviews the development of the Ninth Clinical Consensus Statement by SIBEN (the Ibero-American of Neonatology) on "Early Detection with Pulse Oximetry (SpO$_2$) of Hypoxemic Neonatal Conditions". It describes the process of the consensus, and the conclusions and recommendations for screening newborns with pulse oximetry.

Keywords: pulse oximetry; hypoxia; newborn; screening

1. Introduction and Methodology

For many years, the education, training, and advances in neonatology in Spanish and Portuguese speaking countries have been inconsistent—although this is also probably true for many countries. In 2004, the Ibero-American Society of Neonatology (SIBEN) was created, with the principal objective of contributing to the improvement of the quality of life for newborn infants and their families in the Ibero-American population. SIBEN is a new society, with members from 29 different countries that focuses on neonatology facilitating education, communication, and professional advancement that contributes to the welfare and well-being of newborns and their families, in order to improve neonatal outcomes in the region. Over the past years, it has been demonstrated that the process of medical consensus could be a way of increasing professional collaboration, as well as improving uniformity in the care given to newborn infants. In 2007, SIBEN began annual meetings of a Clinical Consensus Group, where we—under the guidance of an expert or opinion leader in the topic—organized several subgroups of neonatal professionals in the Ibero-American region. Each subgroup critically reviews all the available literature in order to find the answers to several questions that had been posed to them. SIBEN's consensus process is the first of its kind in the region. It has led to active and collaborative participation of Ibero-American neonatologists of 19 countries and has significantly improved education of all participants. At SIBEN, we believe that the critical review and summary of available clinical data as well as the recommendations made by the SIBEN consensus contribute to consistent best practice for newborn care and develops a useful foundation and valuable model to reduce the gaps in knowledge and the clinical care every newborn baby receives in in this region, thus decreasing the disparity in the care provided and improving short and long-term outcomes. Several important neonatal topics, all relevant to neonatal clinical practice, have been covered so far by SIBEN's clinical consensus including patent ductus arteriosus (PDA), hemodynamic management, bronchopulmonary dysplasia (BPD), hematology, nutrition, persistent pulmonary hypertension of the newborn (PPHN), and hypoxic ischemic encephalopathy, which have been published in consensus statements and peer reviewed journals. This paper is a summary of SIBEN's consensus statement on newborn screening with pulse oximetry.

2. Background on Screening for Congenital Heart Disease

The prevalence, epidemiology, and impact of delay in the diagnosis of CHD have been described in several publications [1–8]. Critical congenital heart defects (CCHD) affect approximately 2 out of every 1000 live births; it is estimated that about 40,000 babies are born with CCHD per year in the US, and 1.35 million worldwide, including ductus-dependent lesions. CCHD represent about 40% of deaths due to congenital malformations and the majority of deaths from cardiovascular disease occurring in the first year of life. It is known that more than 30% of CCHD deaths have been attributed to errors in diagnosis or late diagnosis [9]. For example, in UK it was estimated that 25% of congenital heart disease defects are not diagnosed until after discharge from hospital, and newborns may become seriously ill or die. It is now understood that prenatal or postnatal examination is inadequate for the early detection of these potentially lethal and treatable conditions. Delay in the diagnosis of CCHD may increase the risk of death or permanent injury in newborn babies [10,11].

In 2009, de-Wahl Granelli et al. [12] published a cohort study in which 39,821 children had oxygen saturation measured by pulse oximetry (SpO_2) in the upper and lower extremities and demonstrated acceptable test accuracy for the detection of CCHD. Ewer et al. [13], in a similar study in 20,055 asymptomatic newborns, reported similar findings and Zhao and colleagues [14] in China studied 100,000 newborns and demonstrated the same.

In 2011, the US Advisory Committee on Heritable Disorders in Newborns and Children Advisory Committee on Hereditary Diseases [15–17] found that there was sufficient evidence to recommend screening with pulse oximetry [1–64]. The heart defects that can be detected early are mainly the following specific lesions: hypoplastic left heart syndrome, pulmonary atresia, tetralogy of Fallot, anomalous pulmonary venous return, transposition of large vessels, tricuspid atresia, and truncus arteriosus. Screening can also detect: interrupted aortic arch, critical aortic stenosis, aortic valve stenosis, pulmonary valve stenosis. In addition, pulse oximetry screening is useful for the early detection of other conditions with neonatal hypoxemia, such as respiratory disorders (e.g., congenital pneumonia, meconium aspiration, pneumothorax, transient tachypnea of the newborn), neonatal sepsis, and pulmonary hypertension. These findings and others were summarized in a meta-analysis and systematic review by Thangaratinam and colleagues [18].

3. SIBEN's Consensus on Screening with Pulse Oximetry: An Overview

Based on the issues described above, we proceeded to organize the Ninth Clinical SIBEN Consensus on "Early Detection with Pulse Oximetry (SpO_2) of Neonatal Hypoxemic Conditions". The concern about the late diagnosis of CCHD led to the investigation of early detection with SpO_2 screening. These screening programs have detected other conditions that also present with hypoxemia in addition to CCHD that would have been diagnosed later if not for the evaluation with SpO_2 [19]. In order to make recommendations for the Ibero-American region to implement programs pulse oximetry screening, 39 neonatologists and 4 neonatal nurses from 18 Ibero-American countries were invited to participate and to collaborate. They worked for several months with an intense and collaborative methodology, and met in person at San José de Costa Rica, in September 2015, during the Annual SIBEN Conference. Professor Andrew Ewer from the UK was the leader and expert opinion for this ninth SIBEN's Consensus. Neonatal hypoxemia, such as it occurs in critical congenital heart disease (CCHD) and other conditions, is an abnormal situation, potentially fatal if not diagnosed or if diagnosed late, PO screening allows earlier detection and thus the opportunity to optimize their management and improve outcomes.

Several questions of clinical significance were developed on the early detection with SpO$_2$ of diseases that present with neonatal hypoxemia. They included:

1. Cyanosis and related concepts.
2. What is hypoxemia?
3. What is hypoxia?
4. What is pulse oximetry, and what are the normal values in a healthy term newborn?
5. What is the hemoglobin dissociation curve?
6. How does altitude influence on the SpO$_2$?
7. Which are the lesions that can be detected early?
8. How should you do the screening?
9. What are normal and abnormal results?
10. What are false positive and false negative results?
11. How should you interpret the pre- and post-ductal SpO$_2$ difference?
12. What should we do with an apparently healthy newborn that fails the screening?
13. How should we take care of the family of a newborn that has either a positive or negative screening?
14. Is this program cost-effective?
15. When should we order an echocardiogram?
16. Importance of the information and participation of the healthcare team—what data should you record?
17. Who should do the screening?
18. What limitations does pulse oximetry have?
19. What role can the Perfusion Index (PI) have during the screening?

The subgroups were tasked with answering 2–4 of the above questions. They methodically searched and reviewed the available literature, then interacted and worked together as a whole group to find consensus for the answers to all the questions. This SIBEN Clinical Consensus Group concluded that pulse oximetry is a non-invasive method that allows the rapid measurement of saturation of hemoglobin in arterial blood that can detect hypoxemia in asymptomatic and apparently healthy newborns who suffer from severe health conditions such as critical congenital heart disease. In addition to CCHD, the following conditions can be diagnosed early with SpO$_2$ screening:

- Early sepsis
- Congenital pneumonia
- Pulmonary hypertension
- Meconium aspiration
- Transient tachypnea
- Pneumothorax
- Other various less frequent neonatal conditions

The early use of pulse oximetry in apparently healthy babies is simple, very easy to perform, fast, non-invasive, cost effective [20,21], and provides a significant improvement in quality and safety in neonatal healthcare. Thus, SIBEN recommended that programs of early detection or screening with SpO$_2$ are implemented in all places where neonatal care is delivered in Latin America. In summary, the early evaluation of all the newborns with SpO$_2$ is a complementary, non-invasive, easy-to-perform, and low cost test that is performed between 12–48 h of life and is of great clinical utility to detect potentially serious diseases in asymptomatic and apparently healthy newborn infants. The universal implementation of this evaluation in clinical practice leads to a narrowing of the diagnostic gap for newborns to increase patient safety and to reduce the morbidity, sequelae, and mortality of these babies.

4. SIBEN's Consensus on Screening with Pulse Oximetry: A Summary

We summarize answers to some of the specific questions and recommendations below.

4.1. Evaluation with SpO$_2$ Monitors and Sampling Sites

Neonatal screening for the detection of pathologies associated with hypoxemia has been introduced in clinical practice in the USA since 2011. Since then, studies and meta-analysis [18] show that it meets the criteria for population screening test, as well as being a tool in the early and timely diagnosis of severe neonatal conditions. Nevertheless, it is still not universally used in Latin America and work was needed to identify protocols. The SpO$_2$ screening technique is very easy to perform, and should be performed in all apparently healthy newborns between 12–48 h after birth (see below) or before discharge. It should be done by placing a sensor in the palm of the right hand (pre-ductal) and then another in one of the lower limbs (post-ductal). SpO$_2$ readings are taken and recorded from the two sites, one after the other (it is not necessary to use two monitors simultaneously). Screening has to be done with both pre- and post-ductal measurements because some heart defects with obstruction of the left output tract may not be diagnosed when performing a single post-ductal measurement.

The published evidence is clear in relation to the quality of the signal. The SIBEN consensus concludes that evaluating the quality of the signal is fundamental to being able to interpret that the SpO$_2$ readings are correct. Therefore, the screening must be performed with a SpO$_2$ monitor that functions in low perfusion states and is not subject to motion artefact.

4.2. Clinical Protocol

Based on the SIBEN clinical consensus, it is recommended that this SpO$_2$ screening method (pre and post ductal) be performed in all healthy newborns between 12 and 24 h of life, or before discharge home if the discharge is prior to that age. If the first pre- and post-ductal SpO$_2$ measurements are both 95–100% with <3% difference between them, the evaluation is normal and the newborn has a negative screening test. If the first measurement is positive/abnormal (SpO$_2$ 90–95% and/or difference >2%) and the infant looks healthy, the pre- and post-ductal measurements must be repeated once more, according to the protocol chosen by SIBEN, described in Figure 1 below. In infants with clinical symptoms or when SpO$_2$ is <90%, prompt admission to NICU and further evaluation should be initiated without delay.

SCREEN ALL HEALTHY NEWBORN INFANTS WITH PRE AND POST-DUCTAL MEASUREMENTS AT 12–24 H OF AGE (or before discharge, whichever comes first)

RESULTS:

- Normal (negative) screen: One time SpO$_2$ ≥ 95% hand AND foot AND <3% difference
- Abnormal (positive) screen: One time SpO$_2$ < 90% hand OR foot: evaluate/admit quickly
- Abnormal (positive) screen: Any time an infant is symptomatic

When to repeat evaluation in 15–30, 60 min:

- ✓ SpO$_2$ 90–94% hand OR foot if newborn is asymptomatic and appears healthy
- ✓ Difference in SpO$_2$ between post and pre-ductal values is >2% (either one higher than the other one) if newborn is asymptomatic and appears healthy
- ✓ If on repeat SpO$_2$ ≥ 95% hand AND foot AND <3% difference: normal (negative) screen
- ✓ If on repeat SpO$_2$ 90–94% hand OR foot or >2% difference: abnormal (positive) screen

Figure 1. Screening protocol-algorithm recommended by SIBEN.

A second measurement is only done if the first one is positive (abnormal) and if the infant continues to appear completely healthy. If the infant has any clinical signs, they should be admitted, as would any sick neonate for any other reason. The second evaluation should be done 15–30 min after the first in order to reduce delay. Furthermore, if the infant was sound asleep during the first evaluation, they should be alert for the second. If the second measurement is normal, the test is considered normal, that is to say that the screening is negative. If first and second evaluations are positive, and/or if the infant has any clinical signs, immediate admission to NICU is recommended. If the infant appears healthy, they should be carefully assessed as described below.

4.3. What to Do with a Neonate Who Appears Clinically Healthy but Has Abnormal or Positive SpO_2?

Do not ignore the test and humbly accept that we may be wrong in our clinical assessment. It is necessary to evaluate quickly, in a detailed and complete approach, every newborn who has an abnormal test result with SpO_2. The absence of a murmur, normal blood pressure, or the presence of normal femoral pulses do not rule out a critical congenital heart disease. In addition, in infectious conditions or other hypoxemic conditions there will be no heart murmur and the other parameters may well be normal initially. If the diagnosis is not clear, other studies should be carried out for timely diagnosis, including frequent or continuous assessment of pre- and post-ductal SpO_2. According to the clinical suspicion, a complete diagnostic approach and may include complete blood count, cultures, blood gases, and chest X-rays. Some will require an echocardiogram, and in some it will be necessary to immediately start an infusion of prostaglandin to maintain patency of the ductus arteriosus.

4.4. Concept of False Positive and False Negative Screening

As mentioned, an infant with a positive screening test has one SpO_2 < 90% or two consecutive tests with SpO_2 90–95% and/or pre-post ductal difference >2%. A false positive result is when the infant is found NOT to have CCHD. This occurrence is extremely rare (<0.1%) if the screening method and protocol are followed rigorously—although it may be up to 1% [22]. If the evaluation with SpO_2 is done before 12 h of age there are slightly more false positives but diagnosis of infectious and respiratory causes of hypoxemia are more common. A false negative is when the evaluation with SpO_2 is normal (negative screening) but the infant is actually found hours or days later to actually have CCHD. As it can be easily understood, a false negative would be a significant issue. Most studies indicate that the most frequently undiagnosed lesions are left sided obstructed lesions with obstruction to the outflow of the aorta (e.g., coarctation of the aortic arch, hypoplastic left heart, aortic stenosis) which are not necessarily associated with hypoxemia. False negatives can also occur when not using appropriate technology. The use of the preductal and postductal saturation difference and the perfusion index improve detection, but they are not infallible either.

4.5. Altitude and Neonatal SpO_2 Screening

This is a topic that was addressed extensively, including physiology and alveolar gas equation. SIBEN's consensus found that, on average, SpO_2 values are not different in the first 12–24 h of life in infants born at less than 2500 m (about 8200 feet) above sea level. Therefore, if screening is done as mentioned and at the age recommended here, the values for positive and negative results could be kept the same. The issue is that the mean normal SpO_2 is a bit lower at higher altitude (93–96%) but with larger standard deviations. Therefore, some totally normal babies can have SpO_2 of 91–94% at >2700 m above sea level. So, more detailed observation would be recommended for asymptomatic infants, exercising caution and avoidance of aggressive investigations in order to prevent increasing the number of false positives. Still, exact cut-off points in moderate and high altitudes are not precisely known to adequately balance sensitivity with false positive rates.

4.6. Care of the Family with an Abnormal or Positive Screening

In the first hours after birth, various events generate great emotional tension. Health care providers should make an effort to decrease this by all possible means. Families should always actively participate in the care of their newborn infant and they should also be involved during SpO$_2$ screening. As this can be stressful for some parents, every effort should be made so that they clearly understand what is being done to their babies and why. Studies have shown that parents who have been well informed are mostly satisfied with the SpO$_2$ screening test and have perceived the screening as valuable test to detect sick babies. In addition, parents of neonates who had a false positive result did not show greater anxiety than those with negative or normal screenings [23].

It is recommended that parents of apparently normal newborns receive written information on the SpO$_2$ screening test. This written information must be accompanied by clear verbal information and clarification of any doubts that may have arisen with the information received. It is also recommended that the screening is performed with the parents present. In the face of a positive result, appropriate information and support is essential throughout.

5. Summary and Discussion

We have reviewed the evidence in a formal process of clinical consensus and presented the available data that demonstrates that early evaluation with pulse oximetry in apparently healthy newborns does easily detect asymptomatic newborns with severe health conditions, such as critical congenital heart disease, respiratory disorders, neonatal sepsis, persistent pulmonary hypertension, and other hypoxemic pathologies. The objective of implementing systematic protocols in clinical practice for the screening of all newborns by early pulse oximetry is to detect pathologies with early hypoxemia and to perform a therapeutic approach without delays. The consensus group of SIBEN, concludes that adequate early monitoring of SpO$_2$ in apparently healthy newborns is useful for early detection of several neonatal conditions which evidence has shown that the diagnosis is sometimes untimely or late. It was estimated that about 2000 neonates died or were diagnosed late each year in the US, and that around 300,000 babies per year die worldwide because of this. The number of undiagnosed cases in developing countries is higher than in developed nations and it is estimated that less than half of the cases of CCHD are diagnosed in the first week of life. The prenatal diagnosis of CCHD can improve perinatal outcomes for certain lesions [54,55]. Recent evidence shows that CCHD detection has progressively increased from 2006 to 2012, but also that prenatal detection is highly variable in different countries [56]. In some cases, the diagnosis of fetal CCHD is made to later see that the newborn is healthy. Repeated prenatal ultrasounds are much more difficult and costly than simple SpO$_2$ screening. Early diagnosis of CCHD in postnatal life significantly decreases morbidity and mortality rates [24].

The effectiveness of screening is also shown in recent publications on home births in The Netherlands [58], as well as other very comprehensive reviews [59–61]. Adding detailed physical examination to early evaluation with SpO$_2$ increases significantly early diagnosis of hypoxemic neonatal conditions. SIBEN underscores that neonatal screening with SpO$_2$ for the specific diagnosis of early CCHD does not, of course, replace prenatal detection or clinical examination but is a very useful complement. Accurate prenatal ultrasound, physical examination, and SpO$_2$ screening may increase CCHD detection rates to more than 90–95%. One of SIBEN's recommendations is that, at the beginning of this screening program each center must use a clearly defined protocol (as described previously) and at least one quality indicator e.g., performing a random evaluation every 1–2 weeks of the number of babies with screening indication (infants that should have been evaluated) and verified that the program has been met 100% of the time. If this is not the case, processes need to be improved in order to meet the objective of the evaluation and detection of all newborn infants. The quality indicators are not only for CCHD but also for early detection of respiratory or infectious conditions. Physicians should be aware that, even though the combination of early detection with pulse oximetry with other methods of evaluation reduces errors and diagnostic errors, some babies can still be discharged without proper diagnosis.

Early detection of CCHD and hypoxemic neonatal conditions not only reduces the suffering of children and families, but it can also reduce associated costs and long-term neurological compromise by not delaying admission to a specialized care unit. This is also associated with significant reductions in mortality, better surgical outcomes, less prolonged ventilation, and diminished potential developmental problems. For all of the above, actively addressing the neonatal screening of CCHD and neonatal hypoxemic conditions can achieve a significant improvement in the quality and safety of health care, as well as cost savings. In addition, and of significant importance, the screening with pulse oximetry in the newborn has been shown to detect hypoxemia in newborns with severe conditions other than CCHD—such as respiratory problems, sepsis, and persistent pulmonary hypertension.

We conclude, together with many other authors, that significant deaths and morbidity can be avoided or significantly reduced if hospitals adopt SpO$_2$ screening for early and timely detection of CCHD and other hypoxemic conditions [46,57–62]. Its implementation will benefit many newborns in Latin America, where it is estimated that 60% of neonatal deaths are preventable [63,64].

Author Contributions: Both authors contributed equally in the research and writing of the manuscript

Conflicts of Interest: The authors declare no conflicts of interest

References

1. Bernier, P.L.; Stefanescu, A.; Samoukovic, G.; Tchervenkov, C.I. The challenge of congenital heart disease worldwide: Epidemiologic and demographic facts. *Semin. Thorac. Cardiovasc. Surg. Pediatr. Card. Surg. Annu.* **2010**, *13*, 26–34. [CrossRef] [PubMed]
2. Reller, M.D.; Strickland, M.J.; Riehle-Colarusso, T.; Mahle, W.T.; Correa, A. Prevalence of congenital heart defects in metropolitan Atlanta, 1998–2005. *J. Pediatr.* **2008**, *153*, 807–813. [CrossRef] [PubMed]
3. Hoffman, J.I.E.; Kaplan, S. The incidence of congenital heart disease. *J. Am. Coll. Cardiol.* **2002**, *39*, 1890–1900. [CrossRef]
4. Van der Linde, D.; Konings, E.E.M.; Slager, M.A.; Witsenburg, M.; Helbin, W.A.; Takkenberg, J.J.M.; Roos-Hesselink, J.W. Birth Prevalence of Congenital Heart Disease Worldwide: A Systematic Review and Meta-analysis. *J. Am. Coll. Cardiol.* **2011**, *58*, 2241–2247. [CrossRef] [PubMed]
5. Oster, M.; Lee, K.; Honein, M.; Riehle-Colarusso, T.; Shin, M.; Correa, A. Temporal trends in survival among infants with critical congenital heart defects. *Pediatrics* **2013**, *131*, e1502–e1508. [CrossRef] [PubMed]
6. Chang, R.K.; Gurvitz, M.; Rodriguez, S. Missed diagnosis of critical congenital heart disease. *Arch. Pediatr. Adolesc. Med.* **2008**, *162*, 969–974. [CrossRef] [PubMed]
7. GBD 2013 Mortality and Causes of Death Collaborators. Global, regional, and national age-sex specific all-cause and cause-specific mortality for 240 causes of death, 1990–2013: A systematic analysis for the Global Burden of Disease Study 2013. *Lancet* **2015**, *385*, 117–171.
8. Hoffman, J.I.E. The global burden of congenital heart disease. *Cardiovasc. J. Afr.* **2013**, *24*, 141–145. [CrossRef] [PubMed]
9. Kuehl, K.S.; Loffredo, C.A.; Ferencz, C. Failure to diagnose congenital heart disease in infancy. *Pediatrics* **1999**, *103*, 743–747. [CrossRef] [PubMed]
10. Meberg, A.; Lindberg, H.; Thaulow, E. Congenital heart defects: The patients who die. *Acta Paediatr.* **2005**, *94*, 1060–1065. [CrossRef] [PubMed]
11. Ailes, E.C.; Honein, M.A. Estimated Number of Infants Detected and Missed by Critical Congenital Heart Defect Screening. *Pediatrics* **2015**, *135*, 1000–1008. [CrossRef] [PubMed]
12. De-Wahl Granelli, A.; Wennergren, M.; Sandberg, K.; Mellander, M.; Bejlum, C.; Inganäs, L.; Eriksson, M.; Segerdahl, N.; Agren, A.; Ekman-Joelsson, B.M.; et al. Impact of pulse oximetry screening on the detection of duct dependent congenital heart disease: A Swedish prospective screening study in 39,821 newborns. *BMJ* **2009**, *338*, a3037. [CrossRef] [PubMed]

13. Ewer, A.K.; Middleton, L.J.; Furmston, A.T.; Bhoyar, A.; Daniels, J.P.; Thangaratinam, S.; Deeks, J.J.; Khan, K.S.; PulseOx Study Group. Pulse oximetry as a screening test for congenital heart defects in newborn infants (PulseOx): A test accuracy study. *Lancet* **2011**, *378*, 785–794. [CrossRef]
14. Hu, X.J.; Ma, X.J.; Zhao, Q.M.; Yan, W.L.; Ge, X.L.; Jia, B.; Liu, F.; Wu, L.; Ye, M.; Liang, X.C.; et al. Pulse Oximetry and Auscultation for Congenital Heart Disease Detection. *Pediatrics* **2017**, *140*, e20171154. [CrossRef] [PubMed]
15. Kemper, A.R.; Mahle, W.T.; Martin, G.R.; Cooley, W.C.; Kumar, P.; Morrow, W.R.; Kelm, K.; Pearson, G.D.; Glidewell, J.; Grosse, S.D.; et al. Strategies for Implementing Screening for Critical Congenital Heart Disease. *Pediatrics* **2011**, *128*, 1259–1267. [CrossRef] [PubMed]
16. Frank, L.H.; Bradshaw, E.; Beekman, R.; Mahle, W.T.; Martin, G.R. Critical Congenital Heart Disease Screening Using Pulse Oximetry. *J. Pediatr.* **2012**, *162*, 445–453. [CrossRef] [PubMed]
17. Glidewell, J.; Olney, R.S.; Hinton, C.; Pawelski, J.; Sontag, M.; Wood, T.; Kucik, J.E.; Daskalov, R.; Hudson, J. Centers for Disease Control and Prevention (CDC). State Legislation, Regulations, and Hospital Guidelines for Newborn Screening for Critical Congenital Heart Defects—United States, 2011–2014. *Morb. Mortal. Wkly. Rep.* **2015**, *64*, 625–630.
18. Thangaratinam, S.; Brown, K.; Zamora, J.; Khan, K.S.; Ewer, A.K. Pulse oximetry screening for critical congenital heart defects in asymptomatic newborn babies: A systematic review and meta-analysis. *Lancet* **2012**, *379*, 2459–2464. [CrossRef]
19. Sola, A.; Fariña, D.; Mir, R.; Garrido, D.; Pereira, A.; Montes Bueno, M.T.; Lemus, L. y Colaboradores del Consenso Clínico SIBEN. In *Detección Precoz con Pulsioximetría de Enfermedades que Cursan con Hipoxemia Neonatal*; EDISIBEN: Asunción, Paraguay, 2016; ISBN 978-1-5323-0369-2.
20. Roberts, T.E.; Barton, P.M.; Auguste, P.E.; Middleton, L.J.; Furmston, A.T.; Ewer, A.K. Pulse oximetry as a screening test for congenital heart defects in newborn infants: A cost-effectiveness analysis. *Arch. Dis. Child.* **2012**, *97*, 221–226. [CrossRef] [PubMed]
21. Peterson, C.; Grosse, S.D.; Oster, M.E.; Olney, R.S.; Cassell, C.H. Cost-effectiveness of routine screening for critical congenital heart disease in US newborns. *Pediatrics* **2013**, *132*, e595–e603. [CrossRef] [PubMed]
22. Oster, M.E.; Aucott, S.W.; Glidewell, J.; Hackell, J.; Kochilas, L.; Martin, G.R.; Phillippi, J.; Pinto, N.M.; Saarinen, A.; Sontag, M.; et al. Lessons Learned From Newborn Screening for Critical Congenital Heart Defects. *Pediatrics* **2016**, *137*, e20154573. [CrossRef] [PubMed]
23. Powell, R.; Pattison, H.M.; Bhoyar, A.; Furmston, A.T.; Middleton, L.J.; Daniels, J.P.; Ewer, A.K. Pulse oximetry screening for congenital heart defects in newborn infants: An evaluation of acceptability to mothers. *Arch. Dis. Child. Fetal Neonatal Ed.* **2013**, *98*, F59–63. [CrossRef] [PubMed]
24. Abouk, R.; Grosse, S.D.; Ailes, E.C.; Oster, M.E. Association of US State Implementation of Newborn Screening Policies for Critical Congenital Heart Disease With Early Infant Cardiac Deaths. *JAMA* **2017**, *318*, 2111–2118. [CrossRef] [PubMed]
25. Sola, A.; Urman, J. *Cuidados Intensivos Neonatales: Fisiopatología y Terapéutica*; Científica Interamericana: Buenos Aires, Argentina, 1987; ISBN 9509428078, 9789509428072.
26. Sola, A.; Rogido, M. *Cuidados Neonatales*; Científica Interamericana: Buenos Aires, Argentina, 2000; Volume 2, ISBN 89872427570-4.
27. Zhang, L.; Mendoza-Sassi, R.; Santos, J.C.; Lau, J. Accuracy of symptoms and signs in predicting hypoxaemia among young children with acute respiratory infection: A meta-analysis. *Int. J. Tuberc. Lung Dis.* **2011**, *15*, 317–325. [PubMed]
28. Niermeyer, S.; Yang, P.; Shanmina; Drolkar; Zhuang, J.; Moore, L.G. Arterial oxygen saturation in Tibetan and Han infants born in Lhasa, Tibet. *N. Engl. J. Med.* **1995**, *333*, 1248–1252. [CrossRef] [PubMed]
29. Laman, M.; Ripa, P.; Vince, J.; Tefuarani, N. Can clinical signs predict hypoxaemia in Papua New Guinean children with moderate and severe pneumonia? *Ann. Trop. Paediatr.* **2005**, *25*, 23–27. [CrossRef] [PubMed]
30. Dawson, A.L.; Cassell, C.H.; Riehle-Colarusso, T.; Grosse, S.D.; Tanner, J.P.; Kirby, R.S.; Watkins, S.M.; Correia, J.A.; Olney, R.S. Factors associated with late detection of critical congenital heart disease in newborns. *Pediatrics* **2013**, *132*, e604–e611. [CrossRef] [PubMed]
31. Dawson, J.; Ekström, A.; Frisk, C.; Thio, M.; Roehr, C.C.; Kamlin, C.O.; Donath, S.M.; Davis, P.G.; Giraffe Study Group. Assessing the tongue colour of newly born infants may help predict the need for supplemental oxygen in the delivery room. *Acta Paediatr.* **2015**, *104*, 356–359. [CrossRef] [PubMed]

32. Sola, A.; Chow, L.; Rogido, M. Pulse oximetry in neonatal care in 2005. A comprehensive state of the art review. *An. Pediatr. (Barc)* **2005**, *62*, 266–281. [CrossRef] [PubMed]
33. Barker, S.J. The effects of motion and hypoxemia upon the accuracy of 20 pulse oximeters in human volunteers. *Sleep* **2001**, *24*, A406–A407.
34. Hay, W.; Rodden, D.; Collins, S.; Melaria, D.; Hale, K.; Faushaw, L. Reliability of conventional and new pulse oximetry in neonatal patients. *J. Perinatol.* **2002**, *22*, 360–366. [CrossRef] [PubMed]
35. Sola, A. Monitorización biofísica y saturometría. In *Cuidados Neonatales*, 3rd ed.; Edimed: Buenos Aires, Argentina, 2011; ISBN 8963252767-5.
36. Sola, A.; Golombek, S.; Montes Bueno, M.T.; Lemus, L.; Zuluaga, C.; Domínguez, F.; Baquero, H.; Young Sarmiento, A.E.; Natta, D.; Rodriguez Perez, J.M.; et al. Safe oxygen saturation targeting and monitoring in preterm infants: Can we avoid hypoxia and hyperoxia? *Acta Paediatr.* **2014**, *103*, 1009–1018. [CrossRef] [PubMed]
37. Dawson, J.A.; Vento, M.; Finer, N.N.; Rich, W.; Saugstad, O.D.; Morley, C.J.; Davis, P.G. Managing oxygen therapy during delivery room stabilization of preterm infants. *J. Pediatr.* **2012**, *160*, 158–161. [CrossRef] [PubMed]
38. Davis, P.G.; Dawson, J.A. New concepts in neonatal resuscitation. *Curr. Opin. Pediatr.* **2012**, *24*, 147–153. [CrossRef] [PubMed]
39. Niermeyer, S.; Andrade-M, M.P.; Vargas, E.; Moore, L.G. Neonatal oxygenation, pulmonary hypertension, and evolutionary adaptation to high altitude (2013 Grover Conference series). *Pulm. Circ.* **2015**, *5*, 48–62. [CrossRef] [PubMed]
40. Hill, C.M.; Baya, A.; Gavlak, J.; Carroll, A.; Heathcote, K.; Dimitriou, D.; L'Esperance, V.; Webster, R.; Holloway, J.; Virues-Ortega, J.; et al. Adaptation to Life in the High Andes: Nocturnal Oxyhemoglobin Saturation in Early Development. *Sleep* **2016**, *39*, 1001–1008. [CrossRef] [PubMed]
41. Diaz, G.; Sandoval, J.; Sola, A. *Hipertension Pulmonar en Niños*; Distribuna: Bogotá, Colombia, 2011; ISBN 9789588379357.
42. Sendelbach, D.M.; Jackson, G.L.; Lai, S.S.; Fixler, D.E.; Stehel, E.K.; Engle, W.D. Pulse oximetry screening at 4 h of age to detect critical congenital heart defects. *Pediatrics* **2008**, *122*, e815–e820. [CrossRef] [PubMed]
43. Ewer, A.K. Evidence for CCHD screening and its practical application using pulse oximetry. *Early Hum. Dev.* **2014**, *90*, S19–S21. [CrossRef]
44. Ewer, A.K. Pulse oximetry screening: Do we have enough evidence now? *Lancet* **2014**, *30*, 725–726. [CrossRef]
45. Ewer, A.K. Pulse oximetry screening for critical congenital heart defects. Should it be routine? *Arch. Dis. Child. Fetal Neonatal Ed.* **2014**, *99*, F93–F95. [CrossRef] [PubMed]
46. Ewer, A.K. Review of pulse oximetry screening for critical congenital heart defects. *Curr. Opin. Cardiol.* **2013**, *28*, 92–96. [CrossRef] [PubMed]
47. Zhao, Q.; Ma, Z.; Ge, Z.; Liu, F.; Yan, W.L.; Wu, L.; Ye, M.; Liang, X.C.; Zhang, J.; Gao, Y.; et al. Pulse oximetry with clinical assessment to screen for congenital heart disease in neonates in China: A prospective study. *Lancet* **2014**, *384*, 747–754. [CrossRef]
48. Singh, A.; Rasiah, S.V.; Ewer, A.K. The impact of routine predischarge pulse oximetry screening in a regional neonatal unit. *Arch. Dis. Child. Fetal Neonatal Ed.* **2014**, *99*, F297–302. [CrossRef] [PubMed]
49. Piasek, C.Z.; Van Bel, F.; Sola, A. Perfusion index in newborn infants: A noninvasive tool for neonatal monitoring. *Acta Paediatr.* **2014**, *103*, 468–473. [CrossRef] [PubMed]
50. Granelli, A.; Ostman-Smith, I. Noninvasive peripheral perfusion index as a possible tool for screening for critical left heart obstruction. *Acta Paediatr.* **2007**, *96*, 1455–1459. [CrossRef] [PubMed]
51. Ewer, A.K.; Furmston, A.T.; Middleton, L.J.; Deeks, J.J.; Daniels, J.P.; Pattison, H.M.; Powell, R.; Roberts, T.E.; Barton, P.; Auguste, P.; et al. Pulse oximetry as a screening test for congenital heart defects in newborn infants: A test accuracy study with evaluation of acceptability and cost-effectiveness. *Health Technol. Assess.* **2012**, *16*, 1–184. [CrossRef] [PubMed]
52. Ewer, A.K. How to develop a business case to establish a neonatal pulse oximetry screening programme for screening of congenital heart defects. *Early Hum. Dev.* **2012**, *88*, 915–919. [CrossRef] [PubMed]
53. De Wahl Granelli, A.; Mellander, M.; Sunnegårdh, J.; Sandberg, K.; Ostman-Smith, I. Screening for duct-dependant congenital heart disease with pulse oximetry: A critical evaluation of strategies to maximize sensitivity. *Acta Paediatr.* **2005**, *94*, 1590–1596. [CrossRef] [PubMed]

54. Tworetzky, W.; McElhinney, D.B.; Reddy, V.M.; Brook, M.M.; Hanley, F.L.; Silverman, N.H. Improved surgical outcome after fetal diagnosis of hypoplastic left heart syndrome. *Circulation* **2001**, *103*, 1269–1273. [CrossRef] [PubMed]
55. Bonnet, D.; Coltri, A.; Butera, G.; Fermont, L.; Le Bidois, J.; Kachaner, J.; Sidi, D. Detection of transposition of the great arteries in fetuses reduces neonatal morbidity and mortality. *Circulation* **1999**, *99*, 916–918. [CrossRef] [PubMed]
56. Quartermain, M.D.; Pasquali, S.K.; Hill, K.D.; Goldberg, D.J.; Huhta, J.C.; Jacobs, J.P.; Jacobs, M.L.; Kim, S.; Ungerleider, R.M. Variation in Prenatal Diagnosis of Congenital Heart Disease in Infants. *Pediatrics* **2015**, *136*, e378–385. [CrossRef] [PubMed]
57. Narayen, I.C.; Blom, N.A.; Bourgonje, M.S.; Haak, M.C.; Smit, M.; Posthumus, F.; van den Broek, A.J.; Havers, H.M.; te Pas, A.B. Pulse Oximetry Screening for Critical Congenital Heart Disease after Home Birth and Early Discharge. *J. Pediatr.* **2016**, *170*, 188–192. [CrossRef] [PubMed]
58. De-Wahl Granelli, A.; Meberg, A.; Ojala, T.; Steensberg, J.; Oskarsson, G.; Mellander, M. Nordic pulse oximetry screening—Implementation status and proposal for uniform guidelines. *Acta Paediatr.* **2014**, *103*, 1136–1142. [CrossRef] [PubMed]
59. Narayen, I.C.; Blom, N.A.; Ewer, A.K.; Vento, M.; Manzoni, P.; Te Pas, A.B. Aspects of pulse oximetry screening for critical congenital heart defects: How, when and why? *Arch. Dis. Child. Fetal Neonatal Ed.* **2016**, *101*, F162–167. [CrossRef] [PubMed]
60. Lakshminrusimha, S.; Sambalingam, D.; Carrion, V. Universal pulse oximetry screen for critical congenital heart disease in the NICU. *J. Perinatol.* **2014**, *34*, 343–344. [CrossRef] [PubMed]
61. Teitel, D. Recognition of Undiagnosed Neonatal Heart Disease. *Clin. Perinatol.* **2016**, *43*, 81–98. [CrossRef] [PubMed]
62. Ravert, P.; Detwiler, T.L.; Dickinson, J.K. Mean oxygen saturation in well neonates at altitudes between 4498 and 8150 feet. *Adv. Neonatal Care* **2011**, *11*, 412–417. [CrossRef] [PubMed]
63. Sandoval, N. Cardiopatías congénitas en Colombia y en el mundo. *Rev. Colomb. Cardiol.* **2015**, *22*, 1–2. [CrossRef]
64. Reducing Neonatal Mortality and Morbidity in Latin America and The Caribbean. An Interagency Strategic Consensus. Available online: http://resourcecentre.savethechildren.se/sites/default/files/documents/2729 (accessed on 30 January 2018).

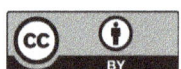

© 2018 by the authors. Licensee MDPI, Basel, Switzerland. This article is an open access article distributed under the terms and conditions of the Creative Commons Attribution (CC BY) license (http://creativecommons.org/licenses/by/4.0/).

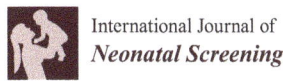

Article

Pulse Oximetry Values in Newborns with Critical Congenital Heart Disease upon ICU Admission at Altitude

John S. Kim [1],*, Merlin W. Ariefdjohan [2], Marci K. Sontag [2,3] and Christopher M. Rausch [1]

1. Department of Pediatrics, Heart Institute, Children's Hospital Colorado, University of Colorado School of Medicine, Aurora, CO 80045, USA; Christopher.Rausch@childrenscolorado.org
2. Department of Epidemiology, Colorado School of Public Health, University of Colorado Anschutz Medical Campus, Aurora, CO 80045, USA; Merlin.Ariefdjohan@ucdenver.edu (M.W.A.); msontag@ciinternational.com (M.K.S.)
3. Center for Public Health Innovation at CI International, Littleton, CO 80120, USA
* Correspondence: john.kim@childrenscolorado.org; Tel.: +1-720-777-2885

Received: 17 September 2018; Accepted: 27 October 2018; Published: 31 October 2018

Abstract: Pulse oximetry screening for critical congenital heart disease (CCHD) has been recommended by the American Academy of Pediatrics (AAP). The objectives of this study are to describe saturation data, and to evaluate the effectiveness of AAP-recommended pulse oximetry screening guidelines applied retrospectively to a cohort of newborns with known CCHD at moderate altitude (5557 feet, Aurora, Colorado). Data related to seven critical congenital heart disease diagnoses were extracted from electronic health records (pulse oximetry, prostaglandin administration, and oxygen supplementation). Descriptive epidemiologic data were calculated. 158 subjects were included in this analysis; the AAP pulse oximetry screening protocol was applied to 149 subjects. Mean pre-ductal and post-ductal pulse oximetry values of the infants known to have CCHD at 24 h of life were 87.1% ± 7.2 and 87.8% ± 6.3, respectively. Infants treated with prostaglandins and oxygen had lower oximetry readings. The screening algorithm would have identified 80.5% of infants with known CCHDs (120/149 subjects). Additionally, sequential pulse oximetry screening based on the AAP-recommended protocol was able to identify a true positive screen capture rate of 80.5% at moderate altitude.

Keywords: critical congenital heart disease; pulse oximetry; newborn screening; altitude

1. Introduction

Congenital heart disease is among the most common birth defects, with an incidence of approximately 1 per 100 live births. Critical congenital heart disease (CCHD) is defined as a structural heart defect with significant risk for mortality without intensive intervention. CCHD occurs in approximately 4 per 1000 live births, and it is estimated that 13–55% of newborns with CCHD are discharged from hospital undiagnosed [1–3].

Screening with pulse oximetry has been identified as a low-cost non-invasive test that improves the ability to diagnose CCHD when compared to physical examination alone [4,5]. Several CCHD lesions are particularly amenable to identification via pulse oximetry screening, including truncus arteriosus (TA), transposition of the great arteries (TGA), tricuspid valve atresia (TVA), tetralogy of Fallot (TOF), total anomalous pulmonary venous return (TAPVR), hypoplastic left heart syndrome (HLHS), and pulmonary valve atresia with intact ventricular septum (PA/IVS) [6–8]. The most widely utilized pulse oximetry screening guidelines recommend initiation at or beyond 24 h of life with measurement of pre- and post-ductal saturations (right hand and foot, respectively) [8]. Pulse oximetry screening in the first 24–48 h after birth has been found to be highly specific (99.9% specificity; 95% confidence interval (CI) 99.7, 99.9), but with a lower sensitivity of 76.3% (95% CI 69.5, 82.0) in one meta-analysis [9].

The performance of pulse oximetry screening has been evaluated in many studies performed at sea level [10], however, studies at altitude are limited [3,11]. Evaluation of the effectiveness of pulse oximetry screening guidelines is complicated due to the small number of infants likely to be identified through newborn screening as many infants with CCHD are diagnosed prenatally or in the first 24 h of life, thereby reducing the potential number of infants with undiagnosed CCHD eligible for screening with pulse oximetry. Furthermore, studies of newborn oxygen saturations have suggested a wider range and lower average saturations for infants born at higher altitude, further complicating evaluation of the utility of pulse oximetry in this population [12–15]. We retrospectively reviewed pulse oximetry values for a population of newborns between 24 and 48 h of life who were known to have CCHD to provide an epidemiologic description of saturation data in newborns with CCHD at altitude.

2. Materials and Methods

We performed a retrospective cohort study at a regional tertiary children's hospital at moderate altitude (5557 feet, Aurora, CO, USA). We queried the electronic health record (EHR) for newborns presenting within the first 24–48 h of life with one of the 7 CCHD diagnoses using International Classification of Disease (ICD) codes in the years 2006–2013 (i2b2; Informatics for Integrating Biology and the Bedside, Version 1.7, Partners HealthCare System, Boston, MA, USA). Subjects included both prenatally and postnatally diagnosed CCHD. We reviewed the EHR for confirmation of diagnosis, pulse oximetry readings, prostaglandin (PGE) administration, and oxygen supplementation data at 24, 28, 36, and 48 h (±2 h) of life. These time points were within the American Academy of Pediatrics (AAP)-recommended window of screening between 24 and 48 h [8]. Pulse oximetry was measured continuously in all subjects with simultaneous pre- and post-ductal saturation values recorded in the EHR. Pulse oximetry values were recorded hourly in the EHR via standard clinical practice upon bedside nurse confirmation of the plethysmograph waveform during the patient's usual calm physiologic state.

In a secondary analysis of the pulse oximetry data, we applied a simulated pulse oximetry screening protocol modeled after the recommended AAP algorithm [8]. Pulse oximetry values were categorized based on the AAP screening protocol: (1) passed screen (no concern for CCHD, false negative): saturation $\geq$95% and $\leq$3% difference between pre- and post-ductal readings; (2) borderline reading (to be repeated at next time point): saturation 90–94% and/or >3% difference between pre- and post-ductal readings; (3) failed screen (concern for CCHD, true positive): saturation <90% in either pre- or post-ductal reading. Up to 3 total hypothetical screens were applied to the retrospective data collected at times closest to 28, 36, and 48 h of life. Data that resulted in a positive or negative screen for CCHD (based on the AAP protocol) were not evaluated in subsequent time points. Subjects with borderline pulse oximetry values at 3 consecutive readings were considered to meet screening criteria for concern for CCHD. Since all participating subjects had a CCHD diagnosis, subjects in whom pulse oximetry readings raised no concern for CCHD were considered false negative in this hypothetical screening. All other subjects were considered true positives. This secondary analysis allowed us to estimate the general effectiveness of the AAP protocol (i.e., false negative vs. true positive) in a cohort of infants with known CCHD at altitude based on retrospective data.

Study data were collected and maintained by using Research Electronic Data Capture (REDCap) tools hosted at the University of Colorado [16]. This study was approved by the Colorado Multiple Institutional Review Board with a full waiver of Health Insurance and Portability and Accountability Act (HIPAA) authorization.

Baseline demographic data are presented as means, standard deviations, and range. Group proportions for categorical variables were statistically assessed using the Fisher exact test. The Shapiro-Wilk test for normality was used to evaluate distributions for all continuous variables. Then, the *t*-test and Wilcoxon-Mann-Whitney test were applied to compare continuous variables between groups for those with normal and non-normal distributions, respectively. Pre- and post-ductal pulse oximetry values collected at 24, 28, 36, and 48 h were summarized as a box-whisker plot showing the mean, median, minimum/maximum values, and interquartile ranges. Mean pulse oximetry readings for various types of clinical support (i.e., PGE, oxygen, both, or none) were compared to each other using the Kruskal-Wallis test due to non-normality of data distribution. Post-hoc analysis was made on groups showing statistical difference. Statistical significance level was set at $p < 0.05$ and 95% CI were calculated for mean pulse oximetry values. All analyses were performed using SAS software (version 9.4; SAS Institute, Cary, NC, USA).

3. Results

3.1. Descriptive Analysis of Study Cohort

Two hundred and fourteen subjects with CCHD were identified. Fifty-six subjects were excluded from data collection due to the following reasons: insufficient pulse oximetry data in the EHR, death prior to 24 h of life, or atrial septostomy or surgery prior to 24 h of life. One hundred and fifty-eight subjects were included in this analysis. The distribution of CCHD anatomic diagnoses between the subjects included and excluded from the study was different (Table 1), but we found no other differences between the groups. The mean pre-ductal pulse oximetry readings at 24, 28, 36, and 48 h were 87.1 ± 7.2% (95% CI 85.6, 88.6), 86.7 ± 7.2% (85.2, 88.2), 86.8 ± 7.6% (85.2, 88.4), and 89.3 ± 6.5% (88.0, 90.6), respectively. The mean post-ductal pulse-oximetry readings were 87.8 ± 6.3% (95% CI 86.6, 89.0), 87.4 ± 7.3% (86.1, 88.8), 88.5 ± 6.7% (87.3, 89.7), and 89.2 ± 6.3% (88.2, 90.3), respectively. Figure 1 summarizes the overall distribution of pre- and post-ductal saturation readings at the four time points. For descriptive purposes, data were also stratified by diagnoses and pulse oximetry readings for each collection time (Figure 2). To evaluate the effects of treatment on pulse oximetry, we compared pulse oximetry data in infants receiving PGE and oxygen supplementation (Table 2). Newborns treated with both PGE and oxygen had lower pre- and post-ductal saturation at 48 h (87.4 ± 7.3% (95% CI 85.0, 89.7) and 86.3 ± 7.0% (84.3, 88.3), respectively, $p < 0.05$) when compared to the other treatment categories (PGE only, oxygen only, or no support).

Table 1. Baseline subject characteristics ($n = 214$).

Characteristics	Study Subjects ($n = 158$)	Excluded Subjects ($n = 56$)	*p*-Value
Gestational age, weeks (range)	38.2 ± 2.4 (29–45)	38.3 ± 2.4 (30–41.3)	0.379
Birth weight, g (range)	2988.7 ± 579.3 (1230–4165)	3071.0 ± 671.7 (960–4780)	0.277
Male gender, n (%)	101 (63.9)	35 (62.5)	0.849
Race, n (%)			
White/Caucasian	111 (70.3)	37 (66.1)	
Black/African American	10 (6.3)	3 (5.4)	
Hawaiian/Pacific Islander	1 (0.6)	0 (0)	0.470
Asian	1 (0.6)	1 (1.8)	
American Indian/Alaskan Native	3 (3.2)	1 (1.8)	
Other	26 (16.5)	9 (16.1)	
Not specified	4 (2.5)	5 (8.9)	
Ethnicity, n (%)			
Hispanic/Latino	54 (34.2)	15 (26.8)	
Not Hispanic/Latino	100 (63.3)	36 (64.3)	0.088
Not specified	4 (2.5)	5 (8.9)	

Table 1. Cont.

Characteristics	Study Subjects (n = 158)	Excluded Subjects (n = 56)	p-Value
Apgar score, score (range)			
1 min	7 ± 2 (0–9)	7 ± 2 (2–8)	0.409
5 min	8 ± 1 (0–9)	8 ± 1 (4–9)	0.212
Prenatal diagnosis of CCHD, n (%)	84 (53.2)	20 (35.7)	0.152
Family history of CCHD, n (%)	18 (11.4)	3 (5.4)	0.361
Genetic diagnosis, n (%)			
Down syndrome	2 (1.3)	0 (0)	0.825
22q11 deletion	6 (3.8)	1 (1.8)	
None specified	150 (94.9)	50 (89.3)	
CCHD diagnosis, n (%)			
HLHS	48 (30.4)	17 (30.4)	
TOF	34 (21.5)	5 (8.9)	
TGA	30 (19.0)	26 (46.4)	
TA	13 (8.2)	2 (3.6)	0.002 *
TAPVR	10 (6.3)	5 (8.9)	
TVA	10 (6.3)	0 (0)	
PA/IVS	7 (4.4)	1 (1.8)	
Combination of above	6 (3.8)	0 (0)	
Maternal age, years (range)	28.1 ± 5.8 (15–42)	26.5 ± 6.0 (15–41)	0.089
Maternal diabetes status, n (%)			
Diabetes (Type I or Type II)	7 (4.5)	0 (0)	0.272
Gestational diabetes	6 (3.8)	3 (5.4)	
Not diabetic	144 (91.7)	53 (94.6)	

Diagnoses are abbreviated: HLHS, hypoplastic left heart syndrome; TOF, tetralogy of Fallot; TGA, transposition of the great arteries; TA, truncus arteriosus; TAPVR, total anomalous pulmonary venous return; TVA, tricuspid valve atresia; PA/IVS, pulmonary valve atresia with intact ventricular septum; CCHD, critical congenital heart disease. * $p < 0.05$.

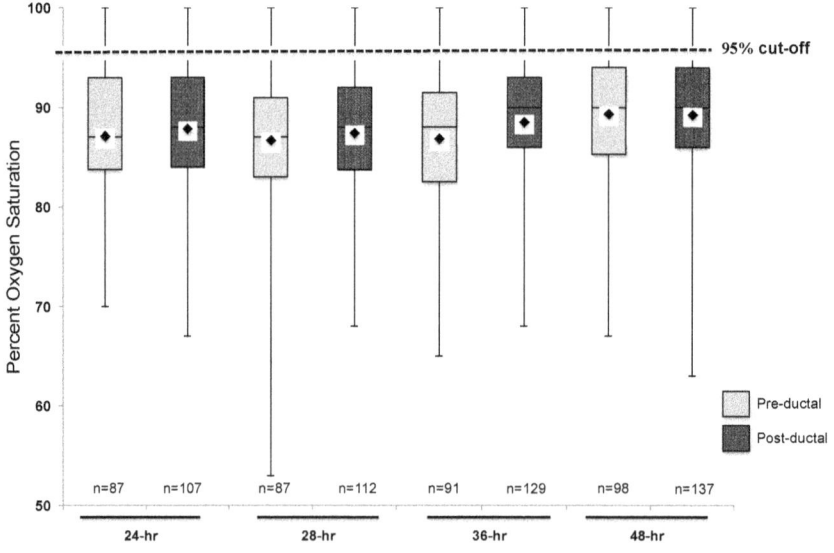

Pulse oximetry readings by site at each time point

Figure 1. Pre- and post-ductal pulse oximetry data at 24, 28, 36, and 48 h of life (n = 158). Mean saturation at each time point indicated by the diamond on each box plot.

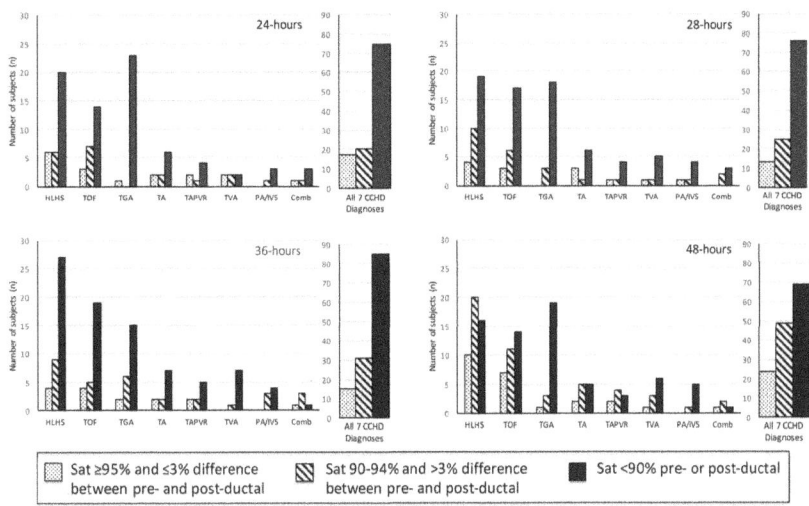

Figure 2. Pulse oximetry by saturation group at 24, 28, 36, and 48 h of life ($n = 158$).

Table 2. Pre- and post-ductal pulse oximetry readings, PGE administration, and oxygen supplementation data at 24, 28, 36, and 48 h of life ($n = 158$). * $p < 0.05$.

		No Support	PGE	Oxygen	Both PGE and Oxygen
24-hours	Pre-ductal	90.3 ± 7.7 (77–100) ($n = 7$)	88.6 ± 7.3 (75–100) ($n = 30$)	86.6 ± 4.3 (80–95) ($n = 14$)	85.2 ± 7.6 (70–98) ($n = 36$)
	Post-ductal	89.4 ± 5.4 (80–97) ($n = 14$)	87.8 ± 6.3 (73–99) ($n = 33$)	88.9 ± 6.0 (78–97) ($n = 18$)	86.8 ± 6.6 (67–100) ($n = 42$)
28-hours	Pre-ductal	88.0 ± 5.0 (81–95) ($n = 7$)	88.3 ± 6.8 (74–100) ($n = 28$)	84.6 ± 7.1 (72–96) ($n = 18$)	86.1 ± 7.8 (53–96) ($n = 34$)
	Post-ductal	90.3 ± 6.2 (78–100) ($n = 14$)	88.5 ± 7.4 (70–100) ($n = 35$)	85.7 ± 6.7 (72–95) ($n = 20$)	86.2 ± 7.6 (68–100) ($n = 43$)
36-hours	Pre-ductal	89.0 ± 9.2 (77–99) ($n = 4$)	88.4 ± 5.0 (76–100) ($n = 33$)	86.3 ± 8.0 (65–98) ($n = 16$)	85.5 ± 8.9 (65–100) ($n = 38$)
	Post-ductal	90.0 ± 4.9 (82–100) ($n = 15$)	90.2 ± 4.4 (79–98) ($n = 46$)	88.9 ± 7.0 (72–100) ($n = 22$)	86.1 ± 8.2 (68–99) ($n = 46$)
48-hours	Pre-ductal	91.0 ± 5.3 (80–97) ($n = 8$)	90.4 ± 6.4 (70–100) ($n = 42$)	89.8 ± 4.5 (81–98) ($n = 13$)	87.4 ± 7.3 * (67–100) ($n = 35$)
	Post-ductal	90.3 ± 6.4 (75–100) ($n = 21$)	90.5 ± 5.2 (75–99) ($n = 51$)	91.5 ± 4.8 (80–97) ($n = 20$)	86.3 ± 7.0 * (63–100) ($n = 45$)

3.2. Secondary Analysis: Hypothetical Screening of Study Cohort

Application of the AAP screening cutoffs to the retrospective data independently at each time point (not allowing for rescreens) would have resulted in 67% failing a screen at 24 h (75 of 112 subjects), 66.7% at 28 h (76 of 114 subjects), 64.9% at 36 h (85 of 131 subjects), and 48.6% at 48 h (69 of 142 subjects). A sequential screening analysis, similar to the AAP protocol, was subsequently applied to 149 subjects as 9 of the 158 subjects were excluded due to an inadequate number of pulse oximetry readings to apply the AAP protocol (Figure 3). Twenty-nine subjects who screened negative with passing pulse oximetry readings resulted in a 19.5% hypothetical false negative screening rate in our cohort. The 29 false negative screened subjects represented all diagnosis categories. The false negative screening rate was 18.8% ($n = 80$) in subjects with a prenatal concern for CCHD and 20.3% ($n = 69$) in subjects without a prenatal concern for CCHD.

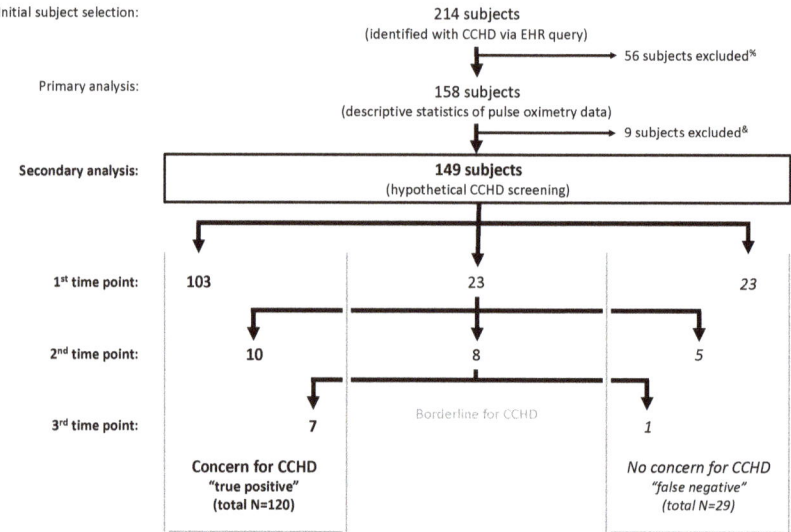

Figure 3. Application of the American Academy of Pediatrics (AAP) protocol to retrospective data in newborns with known CCHD ($n = 149$) results in 120 true positive screens and 80.5% sensitivity. % Exclusion criteria: insufficient pulse oximetry data in the electronic health record (EHR), death prior to 24 h of life, atrial septostomy or surgery prior to 24 h of life. & Inadequate number of pulse oximetry readings to complete the AAP protocol.

4. Discussion

In this study, we report mean pulse oximetry readings in a cohort of newborns with CCHD at altitude and thereby demonstrate the expected hypoxemia of the seven targeted CCHD diagnoses. Prior studies of newborn oxygen saturations have suggested a wider range and lower average saturations for infants born at higher altitude compared to those born at sea level [3,13,15]. We demonstrate in our cohort of infants at moderate altitude with the seven CCHD diagnoses targeted by the AAP (HLHS, TGA, TA, TAPVR, TVA, PA/IVS), that the mean pulse oximetry values are lower than recommended cutoffs for newborn screening. Wright and colleagues [3] evaluated the pulse oximetry screening protocol at 5557 feet (1694 m) and reported a mean pre-ductal saturation of 97.2% (±1.9) and a post-ductal saturation of 97.2% (±2.1) in 1003 healthy newborns at approximately 24 h of life (23.8 ± 2.3 h of life, mean ± SD), similar to what would be expected in a healthy newborn cohort at sea level and significantly higher than our cohort of infants with CCHD. Another study performed at a similar altitude demonstrated lower mean saturations of 92% and 93%, at 24 and 48 h, respectively [12]. Additionally, despite similar average saturation measurements, Wright et al. demonstrated a higher rate of screen failure. This variability certainly supports the need for further study of oxygen saturation and the screening protocol at moderate altitude.

In a secondary analysis we evaluated the hypothetical effectiveness of a sequential pulse oximetry screening protocol similar to the AAP-recommended protocol by application in a population of infants with known CCHD. By evaluating a cohort with known CCHD, we were able to demonstrate a 19.5% false negative screening rate, or a true positive screen capture rate of 80.5%, at moderate altitude. Ailes and colleagues sought to address the difficulties in studying this rare disease by simulation of the population [17] and we present an alternative strategy that yields comparable findings. Our findings are comparable to the true positive screening rate found by Thangaratinam and colleagues [18], who performed a meta-analysis in 2012 of 13 studies at sea level evaluating pulse oximetry screening and calculated an overall sensitivity of 76.5% in screening for CCHD. Further, our retrospective evaluation revealed a similar sensitivity to that of two other large prospective studies (65.5% and 75%) [19,20]. Notably, the retrospective study design allowed us to perform this evaluation in a relatively large cohort of patients with CCHD that has not yet been achievable with a prospective study design [18].

Evaluations of pulse oximetry screening of neonates supported in the intensive care unit have raised concerns for increased false positive rates, issues with oxygen supplementation, and the appropriate timing of screening [21–24]. Additionally, a study performed by Lueth and colleagues evaluated a modification to the AAP-recommended screening protocol with transient oxygen supplementation in newborns at moderate altitude. Their intent was to replicate sea-level atmospheric oxygen tension and induce pulmonary vasodilatation to potentiate the neonatal transition [11]. This group found an increase in specificity of screening with a reduction in false positive screens by providing transient supplemental oxygen to newborns with an indeterminate or borderline first screen at moderate altitude [11]. Because low oxygen saturation in CCHD is primarily caused by shunting of de-oxygenated blood to the systemic circulation, oxygen supplementation in clinical practice does not typically normalize the percent saturation to greater than 95% in hypoxemic CCHD. It is difficult to know to what degree oxygen supplementation resulted in an increase in pulse oximetry reading in our study; however, we found no difference in mean oxygen saturation between patients with CCHD treated with supplemental oxygen versus those without supplemental oxygen. Nevertheless, Table 2 shows the range of saturations in both subjects receiving oxygen and those with no support exceeding 95%. Of the 29 false negative subjects in our study, 15 received supplemental oxygen at one or more pulse oximetry readings (14 did not receive oxygen supplementation). It is certainly possible that removal of oxygen support in the subjects in our study with CCHD would induce further hypoxemia and increase the specificity of the screening test, however, we are unable to make this assessment from the data gathered. This question requires further investigation and the effect of oxygen supplementation on the screening protocol remains unclear. Our mean saturation data do provide some support to the findings of Lueth and colleagues suggesting that oxygen supplementation may not have a negative impact on the sensitivity of pulse oximetry screening for CCHD in newborns. We would not advocate for screening of hypoxemic newborns on oxygen supplementation in the intensive care unit at this time as this is not the intent of the screening guideline [6], however, the findings of this study may inform discussion regarding the timing and process for screening of well infants born at moderate-high altitude who frequently require supplemental oxygen therapy in the first days and weeks of life [13,25]. Certainly, any consideration of pulse oximetry screening for CCHD in the context of supplemental oxygen should be taken with scrutiny both of the patient physiology and use of the screening protocol guideline.

Our retrospective application of the AAP screening protocol did not allow us to exactly replicate the timing of the AAP screening protocol (three screens separated by 1 h each). In addition, the AAP screening protocol is meant to evaluate asymptomatic newborns not presenting in the first 24 h of life, whereas we studied newborns diagnosed with known CCHD. We identify both of these as limitations to this study, however, we used this cohort of infants with known CCHD to estimate the sensitivity of the screening protocol. Further, our retrospective approach resulted in 158 subjects while the very large prospective studies yielded 24–29 subjects with congenital heart disease after screening 20,000–40,000 newborns [18]. Certainly, a future direction will be to apply this study design to a larger cohort of infants with CCHD. An additional limitation is that we found a difference in CCHD diagnoses between the subjects included in the study when compared to those excluded. A disproportionate number of the subjects with transposition of the great arteries were excluded because of atrial septostomy performed before 24 h of life (commonly required for infants with TGA). This may suggest that our cohort of subjects is not representative of the general population of newborns with CCHD, however, newborns requiring atrial septostomy early in life are more likely to present in extremis and not require pulse oximetry screening to identify disease. Finally, this retrospective assessment was dependent on the EHR with pulse oximetry readings that were subject to measurement and recording error from the bedside care provider. These values were not taken for formal screening or research purposes, rather, the readings were collected as a part of routine clinical care. However, these subjects all received hourly oximetry readings recorded in the EHR and the standard is for validation and confirmation by a bedside nurse with interpretation of the waveform when the infants were calm. We identify this limitation to the study design and that of measurement and documentation error by the clinical care team in the EHR. Finally, we applied the screening protocol to newborns who received PGE, oxygen, or both PGE and oxygen, to allow comparison with those who did not receive either PGE or oxygen. We recognize the contribution of both PGE and supplemental oxygen in the interpretation of subjects' pulse oximetry data; however, our results suggest that even when oxygen and PGE were administered the infants still had pulse oximetry values that were low and the therapy did not change the outcome of screening with pulse oximetry in these newborns.

We present the first report evaluating the oxygen saturations of a cohort of infants with known CCHD at moderate altitude. Additionally, we present the results of a hypothetical AAP-recommended pulse oximetry screening protocol in this same cohort. We also found that oxygen supplementation did not impact the ability of the screening protocol to identify CCHD in this cohort, which adds to the consideration of screening in neonatal intensive care units and at higher altitudes. We cannot assess the false positive rate of screening at moderate altitude with our cohort and encourage continued efforts for large population-based studies to evaluate pulse oximetry screening for CCHD.

Author Contributions: J.S.K. designed the study, performed data extraction, interpreted data, and was the primary author of the manuscript. M.W.A. performed data extraction, statistical analysis, and revised the manuscript. M.K.S. was the secondary mentor on the project, interpreted data, and revised the manuscript. C.M.R. was the primary mentor on the project, designed the study, interpreted data, and revised the manuscript. All authors approved the final manuscript as submitted and agree to be accountable for all aspects of work.

Funding: This research received no external funding.

Conflicts of Interest: Sontag has received grants from the National Institutes of Heart Lung and Blood Disorders, the Health Services and Resources Administration, and the Cystic Fibrosis Foundation. Kim, Ariefdjohan, and Rausch declare that they have no conflicts of interest.

References

1. Hoffman, J.I.E. It Is Time for Routine Neonatal Screening by Pulse Oximetry. *Neonatology* **2011**, *99*, 1–9. [CrossRef] [PubMed]
2. Wren, C.; Richmond, S.; Donaldson, L. Presentation of Congenital Heart Disease in Infancy: Implications for Routine Examination. *Arch. Dis. Child. Fetal Neonatal Ed.* **1999**, *80*, F49–F53. [CrossRef] [PubMed]
3. Wright, J.; Kohn, M.; Niermeyer, S.; Rausch, C.M. Feasibility of Critical Congenital Heart Disease Newborn Screening at Moderate Altitude. *Pediatrics* **2014**, *133*, e561–e569. [CrossRef] [PubMed]
4. Peterson, C.; Grosse, S.D.; Oster, M.E.; Olney, R.S.; Cassell, C.H. Cost-Effectiveness of Routine Screening for Critical Congenital Heart Disease in US Newborns. *Pediatrics* **2013**, *132*, e595–e603. [CrossRef] [PubMed]
5. Mahle, W.T.; Newburger, J.W.; Matherne, G.P.; Smith, F.C.; Hoke, T.R.; Koppel, R.; Gidding, S.S.; Beekman, R.H.; Grosse, S.D. Role of Pulse Oximetry in Examining Newborns for Congenital Heart Disease: A Scientific Statement from the AHA and AAP. *Pediatrics* **2009**, *124*, 823–836. [CrossRef] [PubMed]

6. Mahle, W.T.; Martin, G.R.; Beekman, R.H.; Morrow, W.R. Section on Cardiology and Cardiac Surgery Executive Committee. Endorsement of Health and Human Services Recommendation for Pulse Oximetry Screening for Critical Congenital Heart Disease. *Pediatrics* **2012**, *129*, 190–192. [PubMed]
7. Martin, G.R.; Beekman, R.H.; Mikula, E.B.; Fasules, J.; Garg, L.F.; Kemper, A.R.; Morrow, W.R.; Pearson, G.D.; Mahle, W.T. Implementing Recommended Screening for Critical Congenital Heart Disease. *Pediatrics* **2013**, *132*, e185–e192. [CrossRef] [PubMed]
8. Kemper, A.R.; Mahle, W.T.; Martin, G.R.; Cooley, W.C.; Kumar, P.; Morrow, W.R.; Kelm, K.; Pearson, G.D.; Glidewell, J.; Grosse, S.D.; et al. Strategies for Implementing Screening for Critical Congenital Heart Disease. *Pediatrics* **2011**, *128*, e1259–e1267. [CrossRef] [PubMed]
9. Plana, M.N.; Zamora, J.; Suresh, G.; Fernandez-Pineda, L.; Thangaratinam, S.; Ewer, A.K. Pulse Oximetry Screening for Critical Congenital Heart Defects. *Cochrane Database Syst. Rev.* **2018**, *3*, CD011912. [CrossRef] [PubMed]
10. Oster, M.E.; Aucott, S.W.; Glidewell, J.; Hackell, J.; Kochilas, L.; Martin, G.R.; Phillippi, J.; Pinto, N.M.; Saarinen, A.; Sontag, M.; et al. Lessons Learned from Newborn Screening for Critical Congenital Heart Defects. *Pediatrics* **2016**, *137*, e20154573. [CrossRef] [PubMed]
11. Lueth, E.; Russell, L.; Wright, J.; Duster, M.; Kohn, M.; Miller, J.; Eller, C.; Sontag, M.; Rausch, C. A Novel Approach to Critical Congenital Heart Disease (CCHD) Screening at Moderate Altitude. *IJNS* **2016**, *2*, 4–11. [CrossRef]
12. Thilo, E.H.; Park-Moore, B.; Berman, E.R.; Carson, B.S. Oxygen Saturation by Pulse Oximetry in Healthy Infants at an Altitude of 1610 M (5280 Ft). What Is Normal? *Am. J. Dis. Child.* **1991**, *145*, 1137–1140. [CrossRef] [PubMed]
13. Ravert, P.; Detwiler, T.L.; Dickinson, J.K. Mean Oxygen Saturation in Well Neonates at Altitudes between 4498 and 8150 Feet. *Adv. Neonatal Care* **2011**, *11*, 412–417. [CrossRef] [PubMed]
14. Bakr, A.F.; Habib, H.S. Normal Values of Pulse Oximetry in Newborns at High Altitude. *J. Trop. Pediatr.* **2005**, *51*, 170–173. [CrossRef] [PubMed]
15. Samuel, T.Y.; Bromiker, R.; Mimouni, F.B.; Picard, E.; Lahav, S.; Mandel, D.; Goldberg, S. Newborn Oxygen Saturation at Mild Altitude Versus Sea Level: Implications for Neonatal Screening for Critical Congenital Heart Disease. *Acta Paediatr.* **2013**, *102*, 379–384. [CrossRef] [PubMed]
16. Harris, P.A.; Taylor, R.; Thielke, R.; Payne, J.; Gonzalez, N.; Conde, J.G. Research Electronic Data Capture (REDCap)—A Metadata-Driven Methodology and Workflow Process for Providing Translational Research Informatics Support. *J. Biomed. Inform.* **2009**, *42*, 377–381. [CrossRef] [PubMed]
17. Ailes, E.C.; Gilboa, S.M.; Honein, M.A.; Oster, M.E. Estimated Number of Infants Detected and Missed by Critical Congenital Heart Defect Screening. *Pediatrics* **2015**, *135*, 1000–1008. [CrossRef] [PubMed]
18. Thangaratinam, S.; Brown, K.; Zamora, J.; Khan, K.S.; Ewer, A.K. Pulse Oximetry Screening for Critical Congenital Heart Defects in Asymptomatic Newborn Babies: A Systematic Review and Meta-Analysis. *Lancet* **2012**, *379*, 2459–2464. [CrossRef]
19. De-Wahl Granelli, A.; Wennergren, M.; Sandberg, K.; Mellander, M.; Bejlum, C.; Inganäs, L.; Eriksson, M.; Segerdahl, N.; Agren, A.; Ekman-Joelsson, B.-M.; et al. Impact of Pulse Oximetry Screening on the Detection of Duct Dependent Congenital Heart Disease: A Swedish Prospective Screening Study in 39,821 Newborns. *BMJ* **2009**, *338*, a3037. [CrossRef] [PubMed]
20. Ewer, A.K.; Middleton, L.J.; Furmston, A.T.; Bhoyar, A.; Daniels, J.P.; Thangaratinam, S.; Deeks, J.J.; Khan, K.S. PulseOx Study Group. Pulse Oximetry Screening for Congenital Heart Defects in Newborn Infants (PulseOx): A Test Accuracy Study. *Lancet* **2011**, *378*, 785–794. [CrossRef]
21. Manja, V.; Mathew, B.; Carrion, V.; Lakshminrusimha, S. Critical Congenital Heart Disease Screening by Pulse Oximetry in a Neonatal Intensive Care Unit. *J. Perinatol.* **2015**, *35*, 67–71. [CrossRef] [PubMed]
22. Hu, X.-J.; Zhao, Q.-M.; Ma, X.-J.; Yan, W.-L.; Ge, X.-L.; Jia, B.; Liu, F.; Wu, L.; Ye, M.; Huang, G.-Y. Pulse Oximetry Could Significantly Enhance the Early Detection of Critical Congenital Heart Disease in Neonatal Intensive Care Units. *Acta Paediatr.* **2016**, *105*, e499–e505. [CrossRef] [PubMed]
23. Goetz, E.M.; Magnuson, K.M.; Eickhoff, J.C.; Porte, M.A.; Hokanson, J.S. Pulse Oximetry Screening for Critical Congenital Heart Disease in the Neonatal Intensive Care Unit. *J. Perinatol.* **2016**, *36*, 52–56. [CrossRef] [PubMed]

24. Van Naarden Braun, K.; Grazel, R.; Koppel, R.; Lakshminrusimha, S.; Lohr, J.; Kumar, P.; Govindaswami, B.; Giuliano, M.; Cohen, M.; Spillane, N.; et al. Evaluation of Critical Congenital Heart Defects Screening Using Pulse Oximetry in the Neonatal Intensive Care Unit. *J. Perinatol.* **2017**, *37*, 1117–1123. [CrossRef] [PubMed]
25. Niermeyer, S.; Shaffer, E.M.; Thilo, E.; Corbin, C.; Moore, L.G. Arterial Oxygenation and Pulmonary Arterial Pressure in Healthy Neonates and Infants at High Altitude. *J. Pediatr.* **1993**, *123*, 767–772. [CrossRef]

© 2018 by the authors. Licensee MDPI, Basel, Switzerland. This article is an open access article distributed under the terms and conditions of the Creative Commons Attribution (CC BY) license (http://creativecommons.org/licenses/by/4.0/).

MDPI
St. Alban-Anlage 66
4052 Basel
Switzerland
Tel. +41 61 683 77 34
Fax +41 61 302 89 18
www.mdpi.com

International Journal of Neonatal Screening Editorial Office
E-mail: ijns@mdpi.com
www.mdpi.com/journal/ijns

www.ingramcontent.com/pod-product-compliance
Lightning Source LLC
Chambersburg PA
CBHW040225040426

42333CB00052B/3371